GW00458585

RECLAIM YOUR VITALITY

A minimalist way to health, fitness and successful ageing

John Metcalfe Ph.D.

RECLAIM YOUR VITALITY

For Susan

ACKNOWLEDGEMENTS

I wrote this book standing on the shoulders of giants. In my career I have had the good fortune to be exposed to, and learn from, the work of many great experts, academics and practitioners in the field of health and exercise science, some of whom I have had the privilege to work with in person. For this I am extremely grateful.

I would like to extend a special note of gratitude to Steve Maxwell for his inspiration, wisdom and sage advice.

DISCLAIMER

The content of this book is offered as general information regarding health, fitness and successful ageing and is not intended to apply to individual circumstances. It does not constitute medical advice and is not intended for use in the diagnosis of disease or other conditions, or in the cure, mitigation, treatment, or prevention of disease. It is not a substitute for advice from a medical professional and should not be relied upon as such. Before changing your lifestyle you should seek medical advice from your General Practitioner/ Physician regarding your specific circumstances. The study of health, fitness and successful ageing is a rapidly evolving one, and although great care has been taken in producing this book, the information it contains may not be suitable, accurate, complete, reliable, or up to date. The descriptions of the exercises contained in this book are not a substitute for one-to-one instruction and/or supervision from a qualified exercise professional/ trainer and should not be relied on as such. The author and publisher disclaim any liability arising directly or indirectly from the use, or misuse, of the information contained in this book.

'Illnesses do not come upon us out of the blue. They are developed from small daily sins against Nature. When enough sins have accumulated, illnesses will suddenly appear.'

- Hippocrates

TABLE OF CONTENTS

INTRODUCTION

Being fit and healthy is right up there on most people's wish lists alongside love, happiness, self-actualisation and the occasional lottery win. In an ideal world we would all live long, vibrant lives and our inevitable decline would be compressed into the shortest possible time frame at the very end. However, even a cursory glance at health data for Western societies suggests that this is not going to be the reality for most; two thirds of adults in both the UK and the USA are categorized as either overweight or obese, and over half of the adult populations in these countries require long-term medication. While it is true that we can now expect to live longer than at any other time in our hominid history, this luxury is often accompanied by a prolonged lacklustre period of medication and degeneration.

A leading hypothesis in the field of evolutionary medicine suggests the cause of this predicament is the mismatch between our modern lifestyle and the environment our species evolved in. What we now consider normal human living is far removed from that to which we are adapted to. On a physical level, most of us are subtly aware of this mismatch, and by looking to include workouts into our weekly schedules we acknowledge that our regular living lacks sufficient movement and physical stimulation. However, the effects of this discord extend far beyond the physical, they permeate our entire lives and affect every aspect of our health.

It is only in recent human history that we have been able to master our environment to such an extent that we can spend the bulk of our time seated and indoors. While there are undoubted benefits to this, we have taken it to the extreme. It is now the norm to spend our days sat in artificially lit rooms, staring short distances at monitors, responding to arbitrary stressors and consuming highly processed diets. We have created a world of disconnected sensation. Foodstuffs have replaced foods, taste has replaced nutrition, digitalisation has replaced visceral experience, arbitrary performance targets have replaced worthwhile work, and gym training has replaced authentic movement. And as a corollary of making our lives safe, we have made it predictable and largely uneventful from one day to the next. We have outsourced food, risk, thinking, movement and fun, and in doing so we have become complicit, sedentary, sanitized versions of our former vibrant ancestors.

The gulf between our natural ancestral environment and how we now live is vast. And bridging the void has become big business. Sales in gym memberships, complex training equipment, fitness trackers and food supplements are at an unprecedented high. Prepackaged adventure activities promise to provide the authentic life-affirming experiences we crave. Yet despite all of this, a nagging feeling of unfulfillment and ennui persists; gym memberships go unused, training equipment gathers dust, fitness trackers see out their remaining battery life in a drawer, waistlines get bigger and prepackaged adventure experiences at best provide a near-life experience.

Conversely, there is harmony and synergy when living in a natural environment. We only have to look at animals to see this. Wild animals move gracefully and possess a heightened alertness, awareness and perception of their surroundings, whereas captivity dulls them. Our urbanized lifestyle produces a similar response in us, yet perversely our captivity is of our own making. Fortunately for us the cage door is locked from the inside.

ABOUT THIS BOOK

This book is about stepping through the cage door and reclaiming our natural vitality. The evolutionary biologist Theodosius Dobzhansky once noted, 'nothing in biology makes sense except in the light of evolution.' This concept encapsulates the philosophy of this book. At its core this book is about using our genetic heritage as a yardstick to gauge current lifestyle recommendations, fitness claims and research findings and ask, 'does this make sense?' It is certainly not a prescriptive book, nor does it advocate returning to a quixotic Paleolithic version of ourselves. Instead we will be looking to fuse the beneficial lessons we can learn from our forebears' way of living with those of modern best practice so that we can live optimally in today's world. This book is divided into chapters for simplicity and ease of reading. In reality the topics are interconnected and interdependent. You are urged to view the content holistically.

CHAPTER ONE: A BRIEF HISTORY OF YOU

It can be tempting to dismiss our Paleolithic ancestors as brutish, grunting bands of Stone Age people that had little, or nothing, in common with us. Yet in doing so, we are failing to recognize the truth that is staring us in the face. Quite literally. We are compelled to point out genetic traits when we first meet a newborn, 'She's got her dad's nose and her mum's eyes,' we enthuse. And of course we know all too well of our own blessed (or cursed!) familial traits: how we look like our parents, and them theirs. Yet somehow we are blind to this deep biological history beyond a few branches of our family tree. The reality is, dad's nose and mum's eyes go way back through the generations for an incomprehensible length of time, all the way back to when humans can first be recognized as a stand-alone species, which in itself was an evolutionary process spanning millions of years.

Of course it is not just about noses and eyes; all of our genetic inheritance has endured the ravages of these millennia. Under selective environmental pressures our genes have survived famines, migrations, conflicts, ice ages, great environmental and social upheavals. Our evolution is a remarkable story, but this genetic inheritance from our remote ancestors - which was meant for us to be vibrant and robust - is now at odds with our modern lifestyle. Humans have been wild animals for the majority of our history; before the advent of agriculture, every human on the planet hunted and gathered in order to survive. Today there are only a few tribes that do so. We now inhabit a world that is far removed from that of our pre-agricultural ancestors. It is a well-known phenomenon among ecologists that when an environment significantly and rapidly deviates from that to which a species has genetically adapted, the health of the species suffers, leading to increased morbidity and mortality. Humans are not exempt. As our environment becomes increasingly domesticated, we are becoming increasingly ill.

The big killers for us are: dementia, cancers, heart attacks, strokes, pulmonary diseases, diabetes, and hypertension. These were not present, or were extremely rare, for our pre-agricultural ancestors. Of course, they had their own killers to deal with. Attack, accident, childbirth, communicable diseases and infection were the main causes of their demise. However, if they were fortunate enough to avoid this gauntlet they often experienced long and active lives. It is not that they were not predisposed to suffer from our modern diseases (they had the same genetic potential as us), it is that our lifestyle has now exposed us to this genetic vulnerability.

OUR FAMILY BUSINESS

Our genetic heritage is rooted in hunting and gathering; it was the only way for humans (Homo sapiens) and pre-humans living during the Paleolithic period to procure food. Around 10,000 years ago there was a shift from hunting and gathering to cultivation. And so began the Neolithic period, which marked a major change in how humans lived. In recent history we have witnessed the industrial and digital revolutions as well as the rise and dominance of intensive agriculture. Ten millennia have passed since the end of the Paleolithic era, and although this may seem a long time, in terms of evolution it is too brief for any major genetic change to occur. In other words, the design of the human body is essentially the same now as it was for our hunter and gatherer forebears. One hypothesis for the prevalence of modern lifestyle diseases is the genetic adaptations that served us well in our ancient past are proving to be maladaptations today.

It is often suggested that the lack of our modern diseases in ancestral populations is because they did not live long enough for the signs and symptoms to manifest. Whilst it is true we are now living considerably longer lives, many of our modern diseases are evident long before our old age. Anthropologists and scientists have researched the health of modern hunters and gatherers and the fossil records of our pre-agricultural ancestors, and the results are interesting. Younger members from ancestral tribes, and those from contemporary hunter and gatherer tribes, rarely show signs of the early indicators of metabolic disease, whereas our modern youngsters do. Furthermore, older individuals from hunter and gatherer tribes rarely show any signs of them either.

In addition, obesity among contemporary tribespeople living traditional hunting and gathering lifestyles is pretty much nonexistent. This is not because they are undernourished; in most cases they tend to be adequately fed. They also display normal blood glucose and serum cholesterol levels and show few signs of hypertension. By a lot of today's recognized health metrics they fare better than we do.

The day-to-day living for hunters and gatherers requires routine physical activity which provides the stimulus to develop physical fitness and maintain health. Contemporary tribespeople have enviable strength, muscularity and endurance capacity. These days we have largely outsourced all our routine physical activity to machines and in doing so we have created a negative spiral.

We lose fitness because we are sedentary, which in turn reduces our functional capabilities, which further reduces our fitness and ultimately reduces our health. We also consume foodstuffs that are far removed from the foods of our hunting and gathering ancestors and that of our genetic requirement. By default, living in modern society compromises our diets and our physical activity. Our Western culture has become obesogenic, a term used to describe an environment that promotes obesity, and only those of us armed with coping strategies stand a chance of avoiding the ill effects.

It is obviously not practicable, or even desirable for that matter, to put yourself back into a Paleolithic environment. And it would be naive to assume it would be the solution to all our problems. It can be easy to romanticize our ancient past as a time when our forebears lived in harmony with the environment. Yes their biology, lifestyle and environment were congruent, but injury, infant mortality and communicable diseases were ever present. It was an unforgiving period in our history and security, as we know it, did not exist. If life was so good back then we would not observe the inexorable lifestyle shift of current tribespeople towards modern living. Once first contact has been made with a remote tribe, there is an inevitable abandonment of their old ways as they adopt the conveniences and comforts of modern living. It is unheard of for individuals from Western societies to opt to live an authentic Paleolithic life. It is simply not agreeable.

If there was ever a time in our history to be a human it is now. We have made meteoric leaps in our health care. Those of us living in developed countries can realistically expect not to die from former killers such as measles, smallpox or the plague. A broken bone is now more of an inconvenience than a potential death sentence. In the UK and the USA we enjoy average life expectancies of 81 and 79 years respectively. We can expect our offspring to survive to become adults and then become parents and grandparents themselves. Yet despite these tremendous advances we have manufactured a situation where we are crippling ourselves with preventable diseases; we have successfully reduced our mortality, but sadly we have also increased our morbidity.

If we are smart we can have the best of both worlds. We can learn from the positive aspects of our ancestors' way of living, and by adopting their health promoting practices we can benefit from the harmony and vitality they bring. Similarly, we should continue with the healthful advances of our own way of life (housing, security, sanitation, health care, social care, transportation and education to name a few) and reject those which are harmful. It is possible for us to create a new blueprint for how to live a healthy life in tune with both our genetic heritage and our modern lives, and in doing so we can maximize our lifespan and our health.

HEALTH CHECK!

Were our Paleolithic ancestors in optimal health? Although many lived long and active lives, they were not necessarily in optimal health. The driving force behind our evolution was to procreate and have viable offspring. As such most of our evolutionary adaptations have occurred to help our forebears survive to meet this procreation agenda, and not necessarily for them to be in optimal physical and mental health. It would therefore be erroneous to use our progenitors' health as paragon for our own.

Fortunately, we are in an advantageous position. Whereas our ancestors' health was compromised at the mercy of the environment and the actions necessary for survival, we now have the knowledge and wherewithal to manipulate our environment and daily actions to maximize our health.

THE SOLUTION?

I often get asked to recommend the single best thing we can do to move towards a modern healthy lifestyle. It is a tough question, and one I have discussed at considerable length with many health professionals, fitness professionals, athletes and academics. The answer that I feel best encapsulates the appropriate ethos is to start tending a smallholding. On the face of it this may seem a rather strange response, but my reasoning is this: if you are tending a smallholding you will have to move in a practical and opportunistic way. You will bend, squat, push, pull, stretch, twist, lift and carry. These are movement patterns that will help you elsewhere in your everyday life. A knock-on effect of being intimate with the process of growing your own fruit and vegetables and tending livestock is you will develop a deeper relationship with, and understanding of, the food you eat. Furthermore, consuming the fruits of your labour will also increase the amount of unprocessed foods in your diet. The highly tactile and olfactory outdoor environment will enrich your experience and shift your focus from the dominant visual and auditory stimuli associated with modern living and awaken your senses of touch and smell. In addition, being outside will boost your vitamin D levels, and the biophilic, seasonal experience will enhance your wellbeing. Furthermore, if you could do all of the above with a group - say, a smallholding cooperative - then you will also benefit from the social nourishment that comes from being part of a like-minded tribe. It is not Paleolithic, in fact it is more like how our Neolithic cousins lived, but it serves as a suitable example.

However, in the context of our modern lifestyles, tending a smallholding is probably an idyll with little chance of it ever being realized. Nonetheless, there are some good practices we should take from this example and aim to replicate in our daily lives whenever possible. Figure 1 highlights the components of a nourishing lifestyle.

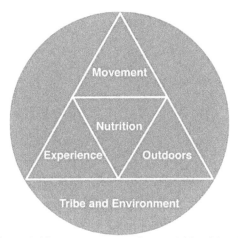

Figure 1: The components of a nourishing lifestyle

With this is mind you should aim to:

✓ Incorporate practical, adaptable and useful movement patterns into your daily living (Movement).
✓ Increase the time you spend in nature (Outdoors).
✓ Eat minimally processed, seasonal food (Nutrition).
✓ Integrate the above into your lifestyle in a way that is autotelic and provides an authentic experience (Experience).
✓ Be part of a like-minded positive social network (Tribe and Environment).

These components will form the key themes for the rest of this book. In the next chapter we will explore why moving more is important.

CHAPTER TWO: MOVEMENT

Movement is an integral part of being a human; controlling this movement is the fundamental reason we have brains. Our brains coordinate our bodies enabling us to perform complex and adaptable movement patterns. Movement is the only way we can affect the world around us. To survive, our hunter and gatherer ancestors had to foresee the future and move accordingly. Throwing a projectile at a moving animal requires complex computation to predict both the flight of the projectile and where the animal is moving to in order for the two to collide, whilst simultaneously orchestrating the body to achieve the objective. Put another way, humans evolved to be intelligent, functional movers.

WHY MOVE?

What currently motivates you to move? Before draft animals were domesticated and wind and water were harnessed to produce power, our ancestors moved because they had to. Hunters and gatherers had to move in order to hunt and gather; if they wanted to eat, they had to move. There was no second choice. As I am sure you are aware, hunger is a pretty powerful motivator.

hunters and gatherers: move → eat

For our hunter and gatherer ancestors there was an inescapable link between expending energy and acquiring it. However, today this association is moot; we are surrounded by an abundance of food that requires little or no movement to acquire and prepare. In this context movement is now an optional activity and is no longer a prerequisite. This has led to overconsumption. Paradoxically, movement is still a necessity if we want to be healthy; if we do not move, we become overweight, which in turn increases the likelihood of us becoming ill.

modern humans: eat → move

We can learn a great deal from the activity patterns of contemporary hunter and gatherer tribes. Research shows that task distribution within tribes tends to be gender specific, with workloads for both genders being vigorous on some days, interspersed with days of low-intensity work. Men will typically hunt for a total of two to three days a week depending upon requirement, and women will gather for a similar period. The workload required to dig root vegetables and tubers by hand is extremely demanding. The children of hunter and gatherer tribes have high levels of physical activity, far in excess of those of Western children. For some tribes, there are also times of large-scale migration in search of food.

HOW DO WE KNOW HOW FIT OUR ANCESTORS WERE?

Form follows function. The activity we engage in affects our physiology, and this was the same for our forebears. Skeletal remains can tell us a lot about the fitness status of the deceased. Bone density can give us a picture of how much loading the body was exposed to and whether the diet contained sufficient nutrients. The size of the sites where muscles attach to bones is a very good indicator of the force capabilities of the muscles (long after the muscles have decomposed). Evidence suggests that hunters and gatherers, both men and women, were robust and athletic.

We are made to function and thrive in a world of lifelong physical challenges in a wide variety of situations. We all have the genetic potential to be vibrant, strong humans, but it is our environment, processed diet and our continued outsourcing of physical activity to machines that has made us the most fragile humans in history. The high incidence of obesity in modern Western society reflects the conditions of our contemporary lifestyle not our genetic potential. If you were brought up in a modern hunter and gatherer tribe with the exact same genetics you were born with, you would be a totally different human being.

Physical activity patterns for our forebears comprised diverse, open-ended, adaptable, in-the-field tasks. Ancestral activity included: walking, running, sprinting, crawling, throwing, catching, climbing, jumping, balancing, digging, grappling, fighting, swimming, lifting and hauling to name but a few. This sporadic and varied movement distributes loading across the structures of the body and reduces injuries and burnout. To some degree this activity pattern is similar to that of modern day cross-training.

The amount of physical activity that modern hunters and gatherers perform is largely driven by the need for food and other resources. As they have no effective means to store food long-term, it is only acquired as and when it is needed and typically supplies only a few days' worth. As such the vigorous food-acquiring days tend to be nonconsecutive, with the time in between spent engaged in low-intensity activities around the dwelling (procuring water, general repairs to dwellings and tools, gathering wood, butchering meat and preparing hides, carrying children and other activities). At face value, their general cycle of activity and rest is not dissimilar to a modern athletic training plan. However, a key difference is their activity is not scheduled months in advance as it is with a training plan, nor is it on a rigid seven day cycle, or repetitive, or split into specific components or body parts (such as the infamous leg day!).

That said, when operating in a day-to-day context, our hunter and gatherer ancestors would have been at the mercy of the situation. Sometimes they would have had no option but to work hard on several consecutive days or they would have gone hungry. One day's hunt or foraging may not have been successful, so they would have had to try again the next day, even if in an ideal world they needed to rest and recover. There were no such things as vacations or retirements. Everybody, save the very young and the very old, contributed. Skeletal remains indicate that our hunter and gatherer forebears were prone to injuries and wear and tear just as we are. Fortunately for us, we can take advantage of our privileged position: if we feel tired we can reduce the volume of our activities and fully recover, and thankfully it does not mean we have to go hungry.

In subsequent chapters we will look at how best to incorporate a hybrid of this ancestral work rhythm into our modern lifestyles, but first let us take a deep breath.

CHAPTER THREE: BREATHING

Everything we do is rooted in how we breathe. It is therefore imperative that you get this skill wired from the outset. Yes, breathing is a skill, and probably one you have not given much thought to. You have been breathing from the moment you were born and you are still alive, so you are an expert at it right? Chances are you are not. In order to develop healthy breathing, it helps to become aware of your current breathing style.

Try this simple test: Take a breath and note which structures of your body you use.

How did you do? If you inhaled through your mouth and into your upper-chest, you are not breathing efficiently. This style of breathing is known as mouth-clavicular breathing and is linked to our ancient fight-or-flight response. When we are shocked or stressed our natural inclination is to gasp air and fill the upper lungs. In emergency situations it is an effective way to inhale air quickly and prepare the body to deal with a potential stressor. Whilst this style of breathing is a boon in a life-or-death situation, it can be unhealthy in the long-run due to the allied stress response. Unfortunately this is how a lot of people breathe most of the time. In other words, their breathing is contributing to a low-grade backdrop of stress, which over the long-term may be damaging their health.

HEALTHY BREATHING
Healthy, complete breathing is effective, efficient and adaptive. It has many benefits, including: greater relaxation, reduced tension where it is not needed, better alignment, better athletic function, improved clarity and state of mind, and the ability to match breathing to specific situations.

Complete breathing
When at rest, the healthy way to breathe is through your nose using complete breathing. Complete breathing involves filling your lungs using both your

diaphragm and your rib cage. Diaphragmatic, or belly breathing, involves expanding your belly as you inhale, drawing air into your lower lungs, then letting it return to normal as you exhale. During complete breathing your rib cage should also expand during inhalation, drawing air into your upper lungs, returning to normal as you exhale. For centuries we have known that this type of breathing has a calming effect, and it forms the basis of many traditional Eastern breathing practices, such as pranayama in yoga.

If you are a habitual mouth-clavicular breather, complete breathing may feel odd at first, but with practice it will become automatic. Below are some breathing awareness drills to help you develop complete breathing.

Belly breathing drill #1
In this exercise we are focusing solely on the role of the diaphragm in breathing. Sit comfortably on the ground (or you can lie supine). Place one hand on your chest and one hand on your belly (Figure 2). Use your hands as feedback. Slowly inhale through your nose into your belly and be mindful not to let your rib cage rise. You should not feel any movement in your chest, you should only feel your belly expand. As you exhale you should feel your belly retract and again you should feel no movement in your chest.

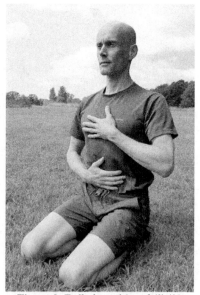
Figure 2: Belly breathing drill #1

Belly breathing drill #2
Lie prone and place your forehead on your hands. Inhale through your nose into your belly and feel your belly push against the ground (Figure 3). Avoid

breathing into your chest. Relax and slowly exhale, letting your belly return to normal.

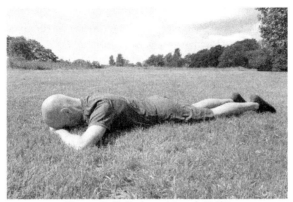

Figure 3: Belly breathing drill #2

Full rib cage breathing drill

In this exercise we are focusing solely on the role of the rib cage in breathing, bringing your attention to the full range of movement that is available. Begin this exercise in a comfortable seated (or standing) position. Lightly put your hands on your breastbone. Inhale deeply through your nose into your rib cage and feel how your breastbone travels forward and upward. Lightly put your hands on the sides of your rib cage. As you inhale through your nose, breathe into your hands and feel how your ribs expand sideways and outwards. Lightly put your hands on the lowest ribs on your back, just above your pelvis. Inhale through your nose into your hands and feel how your ribs move backwards. Breathe deeply for several breaths and focus on combining these three rib movements, expanding the volume of your rib cage as you inhale and allowing it to return as you exhale.

Complete Breathing drill

In this exercise we are focusing on the combined roles of the diaphragm and rib cage in breathing. Begin this exercise in a comfortable seated position, ideally crossed legged on the ground. Sit up straight and elongate your spine. Gaze with a soft focus at an object in front of you. Exhale through your nose. Slowly inhale (for a count of five) through your nose first into your lower-belly, then your mid-belly and then up into your rib cage. Be aware of the structures of your body involved during inhalation. Slowly exhale through your nose for a count of five, reversing the process, letting your rib cage then your diaphragm return to normal. Practice this exercise for around 10 minutes at a time.

Breath awareness

Simply becoming aware of your breathing is often enough to make vast improvements. Throughout the day try and become aware of your breath. Which structures are you using to breathe? Does focusing on your breath make you feel calmer? Pay attention to your breathing whenever you get the opportunity.

Breathing whilst active

Wouldn't it be good to feel calm and relaxed whilst being active? There is little chance of this happening if you are gasping for air using your mouth and upper chest. Breathing this way taps into our ancestral fight-or-flight response and makes the activity feel stressful. You should also avoid the temptation to hold your breath during exertion as this can be harmful to your health. Instead, aim to use nasal-complete breathing even when you are active. At first you will probably have to reduce the intensity of your activity in order to maintain nasal breathing, but it will not be long before you will be back to your previous level. During vigorous activity it is fine to exhale through your mouth, but you should always aim to inhale through your nose.

ANATOMICALLY MATCHED BREATHING

Breathing occurs due to changes in the volume and pressure of the thoracic cavity. When you increase the volume of your thorax the pressure is reduced and air is drawn in (inhalation). When you reduce the volume of your thorax the pressure increases and air is expelled (exhalation). Anatomically matched breathing is when you match your breathing with the corresponding physical movement. For example, when moving into a forward bend the volume of your thorax is naturally reduced, so it makes sense to match this with an exhalation. When returning to standing, the volume of your thorax is expanding, so it makes sense to match this with an inhalation.

As you synchronize your breath with your movement the exercise will flow, and you should notice how less stressful it seems. I am convinced that mouth-clavicular breathing is the reason why people are not motivated to exercise; it makes the experience stressful and unappealing. When you switch to nasal-complete breathing, you will feel calmer and more relaxed, and you will enjoy being active. In the following chapter we will explore how this enjoyable activity should be integrated into your healthy lifestyle.

CHAPTER FOUR: PHYSICAL ACTIVITY REBOOT

In this chapter we will look to redefine the traditional physical activity, exercise and training paradigms that pervade the modern health and fitness culture. We will establish a more enjoyable, realistic and practical way of developing long-term fitness and optimal health.

PHYSICAL ACTIVITY, EXERCISE AND TRAINING

Physical activity is anything that requires muscular effort, and as such refers to all movement. It is only because our modern culture mandates that we outsource physical activity to machines that the term exercise has any contextual meaning. It is highly unlikely that our Paleolithic ancestors performed anything resembling today's workouts.

In an ideal world all of our physical activity requirements would be met by our day-to-day living, and like our Paleolithic ancestors we would have enviable strength, muscularity and endurance capacity. However, even with the best intentions it is highly unlikely that our modern way of living is going to provide sufficient physical stimulation for this to be the case. As such, supplementary physical activity is required. We will refer to this additional prescription as exercise. It is worth noting here that exercise is only used to address the shortfall: you should always aim to get the vast majority of your physical activity from your day-to-day living.

For our purposes, the goal of exercise is to develop the following aspects: (i) muscular strength, (ii) muscular endurance, (iii) cardiovascular endurance, (iv) mobility and (v) injury resistance. While each of these outcomes can be addressed by different training modalities, resistance training is the only one that develops them all. In other words, if done properly, resistance training is the most efficient form of exercise.

OPERATIONAL DEFINITIONS

i) Muscular strength is the force or tension that your muscles can exert.

ii) Muscular endurance is the ability of your muscles to perform repeated contractions, or static contractions against a resistance for a period of time.

iii) Cardiovascular endurance is the ability of your heart, blood vessels and blood to supply oxygen and nutrients to your working muscles and remove waste and by-products.

iv) Mobility is your ability to actively move a joint through its range of motion. This is distinct from flexibility which is concerned with passive range of motion.

v) Injury resistance is concerned with developing structures and movement patterns that reduce the likelihood of sustaining acute and chronic injuries.

Before we continue, it is important to establish the difference between exercise and recreation. Recreation (which includes sport) is what we do in our leisure time for fun. It does not necessarily address all the objectives of exercise listed above, and in many cases, recreation requires specialization and an overemphasis on only one or two of the above objectives. Furthermore, recreation often comes with the acceptance, or even expectation, that you might get injured while participating. In contrast, under no circumstances should you get injured while exercising. If you do, you are doing it wrong!

Exercise places stress on your body, and exercise stress is hormetic. This means that increasing the dose of exercise is beneficial to health, but only up to a point, beyond which it can become harmful (we observe a similar effect with dark chocolate!). Later we shall see how excess stress is a key contributor to ageing. To mitigate this ageing effect, we will adopt a minimalistic approach to exercise and only do the minimum required to get the most benefit. Put another way, we will not be exercising for exercising's sake.

Figure 4 illustrates an ideal physical activity profile for any given week and acts as a good rule of thumb. The vast majority of your physical activity should come from walking and movement. This is an all day, every day goal and you should take every opportunity to walk and move throughout each day.

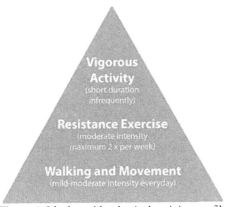

Figure 4: Ideal weekly physical activity profile

We noted earlier that even if you do reclaim as much activity as you can it is highly likely that there will still be a physical activity shortfall and your weekly quota will not match up to that of our ancestral requirement. To address this, you will need to supplement your walking and movement with one, maybe two, resistance exercise sessions each week. In addition, you should also include a few brief bouts of vigorous activity (Figure 4). In the following chapters we look at these aspects in more depth.

CHAPTER FIVE: WALKING AND RUNNING

In the previous chapter we noted how walking should make up the majority of our physical activity profile. This is great news because almost everyone can walk which means we already have the prerequisite skill to get the majority of our movement profile covered.

WALKING

Our erect bipedal gait is unique in the animal kingdom and has been an essential skill for human survival. Our upright curved spine, elevated skull and economic metabolism mean we are ideally suited to walking. However, this style of locomotion means our brains are transported in an elevated position, a position that makes it highly vulnerable if we fall. To prevent falling, our locomotion must provide stability and control as we travel and change direction. These challenges are met via a highly adaptive control system with continual feedback and feedforward messages being sent and interpreted from bottom-up and top-down processes.

Thankfully this instantaneous, functional coordination of our physiology is going on in the background freeing us up to perform other tasks during locomotion. Think about the other complex tasks you often do whilst walking, such as holding a conversation, or following directions and reading a map. This process becomes an even more complicated and wonderful feat when we run, sprint, skip, hop, bound and carry uneven loads. And what's more, you taught yourself all of this when you were just an infant!

WALK BEFORE YOU RUN

When conditions are safe, walk barefoot, or at least in stocking feet, as often as you can. Make sure the area is free from objects that you might stub your toes on, or sharp objects that might cut your feet. Indoors is a good start. There are many arguments for and against running barefoot, some of which we will address later in this book. Indeed, at this stage I would advise you not to run barefoot just yet. However, walking around barefoot is a good practice to get into for several reasons:

1) Healthier feet. The structural integrity of your feet will respond to exercise just like any other body part. The muscles, tendons, ligaments, bones and joints of your feet will weaken if they are not used. Wearing cushioned shoes limits the stresses on these structures and as a result they wither and become prone to injury. Going barefoot rectifies these issues making your feet strong and robust. Walking barefoot will also increase the blood circulation to your feet and legs.

2) Improved balance. Your feet are ticklish because there are a large number of nerve endings in the sole of each foot. These nerves are not there just for tickling, they also provide a large amount of proprioceptive information to the central nervous system regarding movement, coordination and balance. Wearing cushioned shoes attenuates this feedback.

3) Better alignment. Most of your shoes will have a height differential from the heel to the toe (termed, "drop"), and it is not uncommon for shoes that look and feel flat to have a drop of 10mm or more. This drop sets off a chain of corrective adaptations which can alter your standing posture and affect your balance. Eliminating this drop returns your body to a more natural alignment.

There is no need to become a barefoot extremist and literally live barefoot. The naked human foot would not have survived the ravages of the environments our ancestors inhabited, from deserts to rainforests to tundra. Fortunately, humans also evolved opposing thumbs and creative brains, and ancient tribes of humans from across the globe independently created footwear to protect their feet from the environment. In other words, footwear is an integral part of our evolutionary past. But the footwear our ancestors wore was minimal such as: the huarache sandal, the moccasin, or the simple fur boot. The soles were thin and flexible and did not significantly restrict movement or sensory feedback in the way modern footwear does.

It is worth noting that there are specifically designed minimalist shoes on the market that have ultra-thin, flexible, puncture-resistant soles with zero drop. You may want to consider purchasing a pair of these.

How far should you walk?
Anthropological estimates of how far hunters and gatherers needed to walk vary somewhat. This ambiguity is, in part, down to the diverse environments our ancestors inhabited. At the extremes there were forest dwellers and there were savanna dwellers, with every permutation in between. Nonetheless, these estimates tend to coalesce in the range 1200 - 1800 miles a year. This equates

to between three and five miles per day, which is a realistic target for most modern-day humans.

However, as we noted previously, our ancestors moved because they had to and it is highly unlikely they would have been concerned about getting their daily three mile quota in. Rather their daily mileages would have been dictated by their environment and their needs. When food and water were abundant it is likely they walked little, but if they needed to forage over a wide area, or they were following migrating animals, they would have walked considerably.

This is a philosophy that you can include in your walking practice too. Be opportunistic and do not be overly concerned with your daily quota. You may not walk far one day, you may walk seven miles the next. View your walking in weekly terms and aim for at least twenty miles. Some days your walking volume may be relatively low, the next days relatively high. This uneven distribution is exactly what your body thrives on. It is the movement nutrition it craves. If you were to routinely walk three miles a day, that is exactly what your body would adapt to, and doubling the mileage one day would be taxing. Whereas variability in your daily mileage will keep your body in a state of adaptation and prepare you for greater distances.

Take every opportunity to walk, and include some bouts of brisk walking too. Over time you will become fitter, and you will barely notice any effort as you walk throughout your day. It will make walking the easy option rather than a chore. To develop your health and fitness further, you can increase the intensity of your walking. On a predictable flat surface, your only option for upping the intensity is to increase your walking speed. Of course, this can be beneficial in its own right and definitely has a place in your practice, but it also has its limitations.

Inevitably as your walking speed increases you will begin to run, which means that you are no longer walking. This suggests that you cannot get further benefits from walking, which as we shall see shortly, is not true. It is also worth noting that walking (and indeed running) on homogeneous surfaces does not nourish the whole body equally; only those biological components that are involved get the most benefit. And if the terrain is always the same, it is always the same components that get nourished and, as a corollary, the same components that get undernourished.

A better way to challenge the intensity of your walking is to move on varied terrain: sand, dirt, obstacles, undulating and cambered routes. These varied surfaces demand more from your joints, tissues and alignment, thus making you work harder. It also opens up more of your body's tissues to the nourishment of walking. As ever, stay safe and start the challenge at a level that is best suited to your ability. Over time your ability to traverse these varied surfaces will become more efficient and your confidence will increase. This is the time to scale up the intensity and try slightly more challenging variations: you can introduce load-carrying or significant uphill and downhill terrain.

In short, do not underestimate the benefit of walking. In any given day there are endless opportunities to walk and you should aim to take advantage of as many of these as you can.

RUNNING

The benefits of running are not limited to locomotion and getting from A to B. Running is an aerobic exercise and can also provide you with cardiorespiratory development and an enhanced sense of wellbeing. Although we no longer need to run to hunt, or to avoid being hunted, running should still be part of our lifestyle. It is an ancestral movement and is part of what makes us human.

Barefoot running

Over recent years barefoot running has become increasingly popular. So much so that it has split the running fraternity in two: those who embrace it and those who do not. Barefoot running is exactly as the name suggests, running barefoot. There are purists who literally run in bare feet, but there is also a subset that includes running in minimalist footwear. Minimalist running shoes have zero drop and they typically have extremely thin and flexible, puncture-resistant soles designed to maximize proprioception and protect the feet from stones and thorns and such like. They also provide a degree of warmth and traction if you are running in challenging environments.

Minimalist running shoes are the antithesis of the well-cushioned, stabilized traditional running shoe that we are all familiar with. Traditional running shoes incorporate a plethora of technology, the purpose of which is to cushion, control and stabilize movement. They also attenuate proprioception.

But the differences are not just limited to the structure and appearance of the footwear; they also affect running style. There are two main forms of human bipedal locomotion, pendulums and springs. Walking is an example of pendulum locomotion; the leg swings from the hip like a pendulum, and the heel strikes the ground first followed by rolling during the stance phase onto the midfoot and forefoot (an upside-down pendulum). This is an extremely efficient form of locomotion. Sprinting is an example of spring locomotion. When sprinting, you are up on your toes and the footstrike is with the forefoot which harnesses the elasticity of the achilles-calf complex to assist in propulsion.

If we view walking as first gear and sprinting as third, then running is second gear. When running, it is the forefoot and midfoot that contact the ground first quickly followed by a light heel contact (to the untrained eye it looks almost like a flat-footed landing).

Detractors of the traditional running shoe note that a cushioned shoe encourages the likelihood of pendulum locomotion when running. This gait necessitates a heel strike which is fine when walking, but when running it is purported to not only reduce performance, but also create large ground reaction forces which contribute to the high rate of chronic musculoskeletal injuries associated with running. Barefoot and minimalist running on the other hand encourage a soft landing with a high cadence, a shorter stride length, and a flexed knee during the footstrike. Interestingly, detractors of barefoot and minimalist running styles also raise concerns about injuries, this time caused by the lack of cushioning when running on modern hard surfaces (asphalt and concrete) and the resultant force that is transferred to the achilles-calf complex.

Much of the barefoot debate is based on anecdotal evidence, however there is a nascent body of empirical studies in this area. Frustratingly, the data that currently exist would suggest every possible conclusion: barefoot running is beneficial, detrimental or there is no difference whatsoever when compared to running in traditional cushioned shoes. The reasons for this lack of agreement between the studies are the inconsistencies in the methodologies and the fitness and conditioning of the participants. As such the debate continues, and probably will do for some time.

As with all movements, the risks of running are likely dependent on the structure and the situation of the individual (for more information on structure and situation see A WORD TO THE WISE in Chapter Six). To suddenly run prolonged distances barefoot (or in minimalist footwear) following years of being sedentary, or running in cushioned footwear, is clearly asking for trouble. Whereas following a correct strength and conditioning programme and graded exposure, barefoot or minimalist running will likely be of great benefit. Many of the world's indigenous tribes run barefoot or in minimalist footwear (often wearing huarache sandals) and this has led partisan barefoot runners to suggest that the barefoot running style is the way we are meant to run. Maybe one day the debate will be concluded. Personally, I prefer minimalist and barefoot running.

MINIMALIST RUNNING FORM

If you do decide to become a minimalist runner I would encourage you to consult a qualified running coach; there is no substitute for one-to-one coaching. As a rule of thumb, when making the transition, minimalist running should only make up about 5% of your running total, the rest should be in your regular running footwear. Then gradually increase the minimalist running contribution as you adapt. (This process may take a year or more, especially if your feet are unaccustomed to walking and running barefoot or in minimalist footwear).

Mini-jumps help strengthen and coordinate the anatomy associated with running. From a standing position, raise your heels off the ground, but do not fully raise onto your toes. Look straight ahead and bounce up and down. Only jump a couple of centimetres off the ground; we are not going for height here, just small, light, frequent bounces. Land on your fore and midfeet and let your heels lightly kiss the ground (it should look like you are almost landing flat-footed). Develop your coordination so that you remain on the same spot on the ground whilst looking straight ahead. At first you might notice that you migrate forward or to one side. Over time you will develop consistency with this skill, then you can progress to switching from one leg to the other. Again, only small movements are required.

To run, mimic this alternating action, lean slightly forward at the ankles and maintain an upright torso (imagine your hips are gently being pulled forward by an invisible thread) and run. Focus on lifting your feet rather than driving off them. Ideally your lead foot should land underneath (not in front of) you with a flexed knee to aid shock absorption. During the swing phase of your rear leg, your foot should pass level with the knee of your stance leg. Your arms should be at the side of your ribs with hands slightly higher than your elbows. With this style of running you should notice that your stride length decreases and the frequency of your footfalls increases (up to about 180 strikes per minute) compared with your old style of running.

Reset your experience of running: Zen running

Running tends to split emotions too. It creates fervour in some and disdain, or even horror, in others. Personally, I love the experience of running. I practice Zen running and enjoy the feeling of locomotion when the harmonics of my footfalls, breathing rate, and pulse synchronize and become one. For me running is a form of meditation. Running provides me with an opportunity to tune into my body and for this reason I never wear headphones as I regard them as a distraction from the intrinsic pleasure of the movement (I also apply this philosophy to exercise). From my experience those who tend to dislike running are mouth-clavicular breathers. Their heavy breathing and grimacing puts them in a stressed state. No wonder these runners want the distraction of music or podcasts.

In Chapter Three we looked at the importance of breathing and how we should always aim to inhale via the nose and not the mouth. This also applies to running. Focus on your breath whilst warming up and use it to gauge your running intensity. Begin at a mild-moderate intensity and gradually build up the pace. If you feel you need to use your mouth to inhale, you are running too fast.

This style of running is called Zen running. Ego is the enemy of Zen running. During the first few weeks your pace will be pedestrian, so avoid being distracted with distances and split times. As you become a more efficient nasal breather, your speed will increase, and so too will your enjoyment.

Unlike our ancestors' lives, your day-to-day life may not require much running. If this is the case be opportunistic and run whenever you can. Even short, infrequent distances are fine, they all add up. Keep an eye on your overall weekly running volume and if the opportunity for spontaneous running has not presented itself for a few days, make a conscious effort to include a scheduled run to make up the shortfall.

The take home message from this chapter is straightforward: walk as often as you can and add in some occasional running. Simple.

CHAPTER SIX: GET MOVING!

O ur ancestral activity included a plethora of movement patterns (such as: jumping, climbing, crawling, grappling, fighting, swimming and so on), and you were probably doing most of these activities without a second thought when you were a kid (lamentably research is indicating that this is happening less and less with today's children). However, like most adults, you have probably lost the ability to perform most of these movements effectively and efficiently. Think about it, when did you last crawl on the ground? When was the last time you climbed anything other than your stairs? Can you perform the full squat with the ease that a child can?

To reclaim your vitality as a human you are going to need to reclaim these natural human movements. Like the recommendations for walking and running, you should take every opportunity to incorporate as many of these activities as you can into each day (with the exceptions of grappling and fighting of course, save these for martial arts classes!).

MOVEMENT IS YOUR BIRTHRIGHT

Phylogenetic movements are those that are unique to a particular species. Humans are not the fastest animals on the planet, nor are we the strongest, but whereas most animals are specialists and have limited phylogenetic movements, we excel in being movement generalists. In 1957 Scientific American published a seminal paper by anthropologist Gordon W Hewes in which he detailed all of the postures that are natural to the human species. There are literally hundreds!

Nowadays our convenient way of living requires little movement bandwidth, and as a result most Westerners no longer need, and can no longer perform, these phylogenetic postures. Sports and gym-based workouts compound the problem by training us to become specialists in uniplanar movement patterns at the expense of being generalist multiplanar movers. Sadly, this loss of movement repertoire means we also lose a part of what being human is about.

If you have lost the mobility to perform these archetypal postures and movements, it is not going to be possible for you to seamlessly integrate them into your daily life from the get-go. As such you will need to set aside some time for practice and adaptation before they can become part of your everyday life. Below we will look at developing the prerequisite fitness for basic: i) squatting, ii) sitting, iii) jumping, iv) climbing and v) crawling.

A WORD TO THE WISE

There is a culture within the fitness industry that arbitrarily labels one exercise dangerous and another one safe. In reality, how safe an exercise is depends upon the structure (physical fitness) and the situation (context) for each individual. For example, squatting below parallel may be inappropriate for a sedentary overweight man, whereas advisable for an appropriately trained athlete. Furthermore, following several months of corrective exercises, the full squat may be beneficial for the aforementioned sedentary man providing he now possess the prerequisite strength and conditioning. Injury and health status also play a role in exercise suitability.

Before you perform any exercise, you must first take into account your current structure and the situation you are in. Addressing these two concepts should help you make the correct decision when choosing a movement and the range through which to perform it. You will recall that a requisite of exercise is it should reduce the likelihood of injuries and not contribute to them. Before you begin, I recommend you seek advice from your GP/ physician and a competent strength and conditioning/ movement coach to determine these two personal aspects. This is an ongoing process that requires continuous evaluation; as your structure and situation change, so does the appropriateness (or not) of the different exercises.

SQUATTING
Full squat
This squat goes under various names (I have even seen it referred to as the bathrooming squat!), but it is essentially just a full-range squat with your heels on the ground. I use the word "just", but most adults cannot perform this movement. The chief reason for this is a lack of mobility particularly at the hips, knees and ankle joints. Prolonged sitting in chairs contributes to this issue as it restricts the range of motion at these joints. Think about how long you spend sitting during a typical day: in the car, at the office, eating, watching television, the list goes on.

The full squat will probably not come easy. In the correct position your feet should be hip-width apart, parallel and your heels should be on the ground. You should have maximum flexion at your hips, knees and ankles, and your centre of mass should be positioned over your forefeet (Figure 5). When you first attempt this, you may feel like you are going to topple over backwards. If this is the case, you can stabilize yourself and support some of the load by holding onto a sturdy object in front of you. Make sure you stay within a comfortable, yet challenging, range of motion.

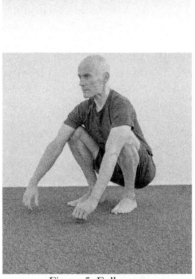

Figure 5: Full squat

Most people quickly adopt the cheat squat position by increasing the width of their stance and splaying their feet. Another cheat is allowing the knees to move inwards (knee valgus) which inadvertently increases the loading on the inside of the knee joints and leaves the lower back vulnerable. Avoid these cheats as they are harmful practices. If you notice them happening, back off and stay only in the range where your correct form allows. To prevent knee valgus, attempt to corkscrew your feet outwards without actually moving them. This helps prevent the internal rotation of the thighs which causes the valgus.

Do not force or rush the process. The correct position will seem effortful in the beginning, but over time it should become a restful and relaxed position. This is how many people from non-Western cultures sit. The full squat helps maintain mobility at the hips, knees, ankles and spine, the very things sitting in a chair reduces. Correcting these factors will contribute to developing better alignment.

Full knee bend
This is similar to the full squat, but now you are balancing on the balls of your feet, with your heels off the ground (Figure 6). This requires less mobility but a lot more balance, so it is wise to hold onto a sturdy object for support at first. When you are proficient in both the full squat and the full knee bend, practice

transitioning in a controlled manner from one to the other and back. Support yourself if necessary.

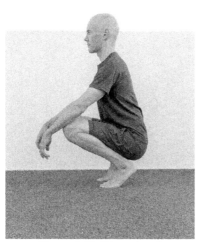

Figure 6: Full knee bend

SITTING

Unfortunately we already tend to do a lot of sitting. Current estimates suggest a typical Western adult spends over half the day seated. Time spent seated has been shown to be an independent health risk factor. And as we have seen, chair sitting is a main contributor to reduced mobility. However, in this section I am not advocating sitting in a chair, instead I am suggesting sitting on the ground.

  There are many different seated positions for you to play around with. Instead of watching television from the couch, sit on a rug or mat and experiment with different sitting postures. Below are ten archetypal sitting postures you can practice:

1) Sphinx pose

Lie prone, propped up on your elbows (Figure 7). Your elbows should be directly underneath your shoulders. Depress your shoulders and stretch the crown of your head as far away from your shoulders as possible (aim to maximize the distance between your ears and your shoulders).

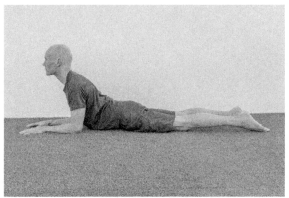

Figure 7: Sphinx pose

2) Lying

Lie on your side, supporting your head with your hand (Figure 8). Alternate sides.

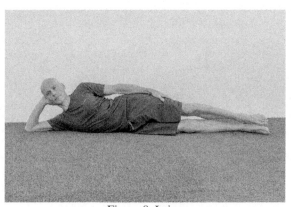

Figure 8: Lying

3) Seiza sit

Kneel and sit on your heels with the tops of your feet flat on the ground (Figure 9). Aim to maintain an upright torso.

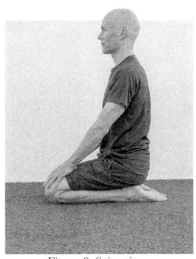

Figure 9: Seiza sit

4) Samurai sit

Kneel and sit on your heels with your toes curled under (Figure 10). Aim to maintain an upright torso. This is a great exercise for developing foot strength.

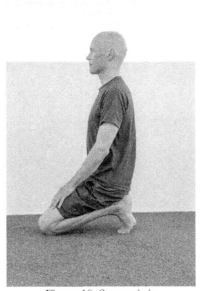

Figure 10: Samurai sit

5) Full squat

Squat down with your feet hip-width apart, parallel and your heels on the ground (Figure 11). You should have maximum flexion at your hips, knees and ankles, and your centre of mass should be positioned over your forefeet.

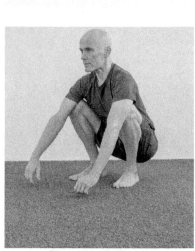

Figure 11: Full squat

6) Hunter squat

This is a combination of the full squat and the seiza sit (Figure 12). Kneel down and sit on the heel of your right foot. Your left leg should be in front of you with maximum flexion at the hip and knee. Your left foot should be flat on the floor. Alternate sides.

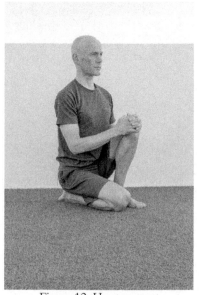

Figure 12: Hunter squat

7) Sit with crossed legs

Sitting crossed legged is good for hip mobility (Figure 13). There are several variations depending on your current ability. Choose one that is comfortable yet challenging for you. Be mindful to elongate your spine and avoid rounding your back. In the beginning you may need to bolster your hips by sitting on a cushion.

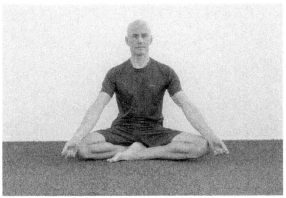

Figure 13: Crossed legs

8) Staff pose (or L sit)

Sit with your legs directly out in front of you and your torso upright (Figure 14). If this is uncomfortable in the beginning, you can bend your knees and use your arms as posts. Be mindful to elongate your spine and avoid rounding your back.

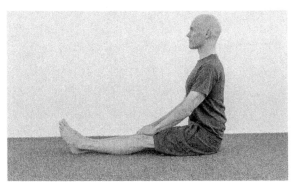

Figure 14: Staff pose (or L sit)

9) Straddle sit

Sit with your legs wide and your torso upright (Figure 15). Be mindful to elongate your spine and avoid rounding your back.

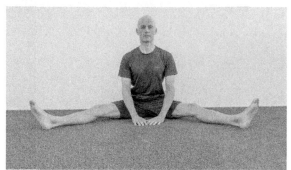

Figure 15: Straddle sit

10) Shin box

Sit with one leg bent in front of you, the other bent behind (Figure 16). The sole of your front foot should be level with the knee of your back leg. Maintain an upright torso. This is often called the Z-sit as the legs make a 'Z' shape. Alternate sides.

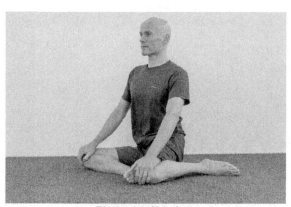

Figure 16: Shin box

If, in the beginning, the postures are uncomfortable, or you do not yet have the mobility you can use your arms as posts to assist you (Figure 17).

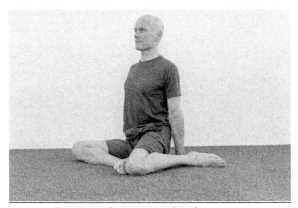

Figure 17: Sitting using hands as posts

Continual sitting in any position for hours a day is not advisable, even the ones noted above. It is the lack of movement that is harmful to health. So only hold a seated position for a short while and then move into another one. (Sitting on the floor is not as comfortable as sitting on the couch, so you will naturally want to switch your sitting postures anyway).

The above seated examples can be performed in sequence. Challenge yourself, try transitioning from one to another. You may need some assistance from your arms at first, but over time lessen your dependence on them so that you can transition from one seated position to another with minimal or no assistance. Progress to getting into and out of a sitting position from standing.

Step-through
The step-through is a movement pattern that has a lot of uses. It can be used to transition between crawls (see later) and other actions such as getting over a low wall (see later). It is also an efficient way to get down and up from the ground. Contemporary research is finding that the ability to get down and up from the ground is a strong predictor of longevity and independence in old age.

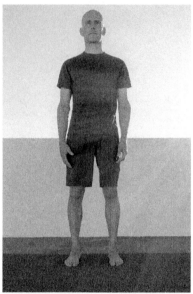

Figure 18: Step-through: Start and finish position

From a standing position (Figure 18) lean over to your right side and place your right hand on the ground directly under your shoulder (Figure 19).

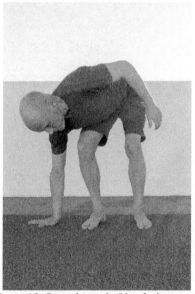

Figure 19: Step-through: Hand placement

Take the weight off your right foot and extend your right leg in front of you. Your weight should be evenly distributed between your right hand and your left foot, your hips and right leg should be off the ground (Figure 20).

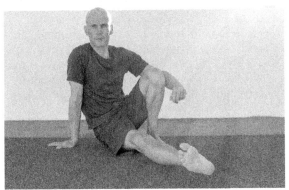
Figure 20: Step-through: Leg extension

Bring your right foot back between your left foot and right hand, and place it on the outside of your right hand (Figure 21).

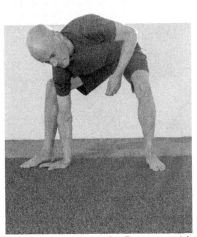
Figure 21: Step-through: Get-up position

Stand up and return to the start position by bringing your right foot back to a hip-width stance (Figure 18). Repeat on the other side.

JUMPING

Jumping is a locomotive skill that all healthy humans should be able to perform. However, you should not attempt to jump if you do not currently have the appropriate strength and conditioning. During the landing phase you will experience forces several times your body weight; these forces can easily expose you to an unacceptable level of risk. It is an immutable fact that it is impossible to jump without landing, so your jump practice should focus first on getting the landing perfected. This is also a good place to start to develop the prerequisite strength and conditioning for jumping.

Landing alignment

From a standing position, slowly raise onto your toes, lower back down and as your heels lightly touch the ground, bend at the knees and lower into a quarter squat whilst simultaneously raising your arms to the front to act as a counterbalance (Figure 22). In this position, your shoulders should be vertically aligned over your knees. Return to standing position. Practice this and be mindful of your form; try to make it one fluid motion.

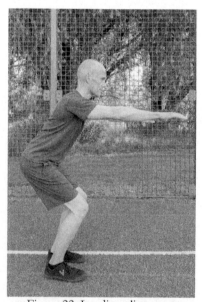

Figure 22: Landing alignment

Once you are competent at this movement, you can add just enough extra force in the upward direction so that, although your toes and the balls of your feet are still in contact with the ground, you feel weightless, effectively jumping without leaving the ground. Once again be mindful of the landing phase and pay particular attention to correct form. This is especially so now there is extra force involved. The controlled action of your forefeet momentarily making contact first, followed by light contact with your heels, then absorption through your leg and hip muscles as your leg joints move into flexion is what helps disperse the landing forces. Under no circumstances should you be landing heels first, or with your knees locked. Use your arms as a counterbalance and once you have decelerated at the bottom position, return to standing. As your proficiency develops increase the jump force so that you leave the ground by few centimetres.

Once you have built the appropriate strength and conditioning and have developed the prerequisite landing skill you can progress onto the broad jump and the vertical jump.

Broad jump

A broad jump is a two-footed horizontal jump. It is the sort of technique you would use to clear an obstacle when there is not enough room for a run up.

From a standing position, identify your landing spot. With a slight forward lean, bend at the knees bringing your arms behind you. Rapidly swing your arms forward and as they pass in front of your hips push off with your legs, jumping forward (Figures 23 to 26). The amount of forward lean, knee flexion and arm swing should be determined by how far you want to jump. There is a lot going on with this skill and the forces your body will experience can be quite high, so start off with short distances and then progress as you feel comfortable.

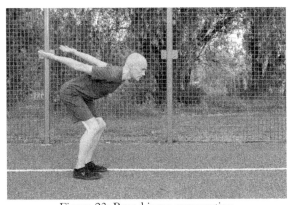

Figure 23: Broad jump preparation

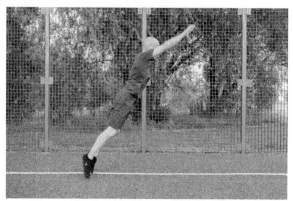

Figure 24: Broad jump take-off

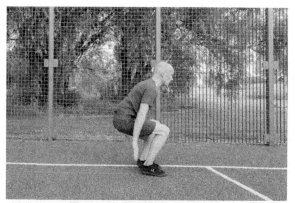

Figure 25: Broad jump landing

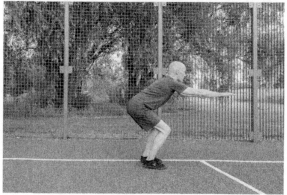

Figure 26: Broad jump finish

Vertical jump

A vertical jump is a two-footed upward jump. It is the sort of technique you would use to touch something that is slightly out of reach, or jump on to a higher surface.

From a standing position, identify what you are jumping to touch (or your landing spot if jumping on to a higher surface). Bend at the knees and lower into a quarter squat bringing your arms behind you. Rapidly swing your arms forward and upwards. As they pass in front of your hips push off with your legs, jumping upwards (and slightly forwards if jumping on to a higher surface). If you are jumping to touch something overhead your arms should be extended upwards and you should be looking at your target (Figures 27 and 28). If you are jumping on to an object you should bring your knees up. As with the broad jump, there is a lot going on with this skill and the forces your body will experience can be quite high, so start off with low heights and then progress as you feel comfortable.

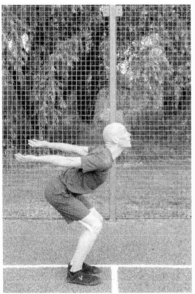 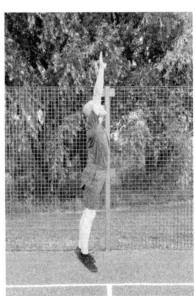

Figure 27: Vertical jump preparation   Figure 28: Vertical jump take-off

CLIMBING

Detailed below are several basic climbing skills. Begin with the one that is most appropriate to you.

Side hang

The side hang is a great introduction to hanging and climbing as it only applies a low load. To side hang stand next to a sturdy vertical post or pole. Reach out with your nearest hand and grab it. Lean away from the pole until your arm is straight (Figure 29). You can modulate the load that you apply by moving your feet towards or away from the pole. Moving your feet nearer the pole increases the load, moving them away reduces the load. From this position you can also perform shoulder retraction (drawing your shoulder blade towards the midline of your body with your arm straight), pulling yourself towards the pole.

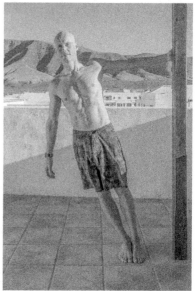

Figure 29: Side hang

Sit-back hang

This is a good progression from the side hang as it helps to develop the prerequisite mobility and strength for the overhead bar hang. Stand facing a sturdy vertical post or pole a little less than an arm's length in front of you. Firmly grasp the post at shoulder height with both hands and sit back with your arms straight. Aim to get your wrists, elbows, shoulders and hips in line (Figure 30). You may need to shuffle your foot position to allow for this.

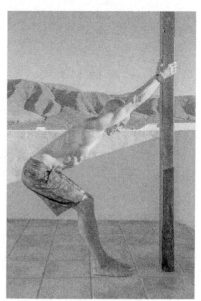

Figure 30: Sit-back hang

Supported hang

With this exercise, you hang off a sturdy horizontal bar with your feet on the ground (Figure 31). This requires a bar at a specific height, or you can use a pull-up bar with a sturdy box underneath to stand on. Grab the bar with a shoulder-width overhand grip (palms facing away), your knees should be bent and your feet on the ground. Hang from the bar and modulate the load on your grip by increasing or decreasing the contribution from your legs. As you become stronger you should be able to support your entire body weight.

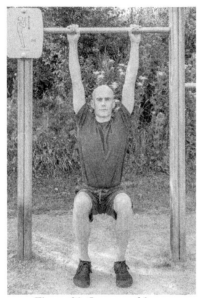

Figure 31: Supported hang

Bar hang

If you have the appropriate strength and conditioning you can progress to bar hanging. Hanging is a key exercise as it is the precursor to many other advanced movements, such as pull-ups, muscle-ups and brachiating to name a few. A corollary of hanging is increased grip strength, which is useful in day-to-day activities. In addition, grip strength has been found to enjoy a positive correlation with longevity. Hanging also develops shoulder mobility and can have a beneficial effect on spinal alignment.

There are two main categories of hanging: passive and active. In the passive variation your shoulders are relaxed and up around your ears (Figure 32). In the active hang you depress your shoulders by drawing the shoulder blades down your back (Figure 33). Practise both. A good exercise for shoulder health is to transition between the two several times.

41

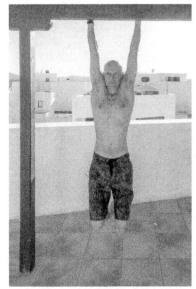 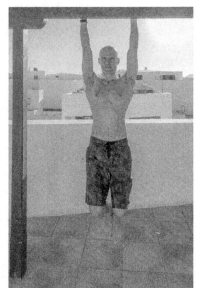

Figure 32: Passive hang   Figure 33: Active hang

Hanging for several minutes at a time is beneficial, but in the early stages increased frequency is more important. By this I mean 6 x 20-second hangs spread throughout the day is better than a single two-minute hang. The focus is on making the action familiar, then once you are comfortable with it you can increase the duration.

Wall support hold
The wall support hold is a great starter exercise for developing straight arm strength and is a basic climbing skill. The wall support when performed in conjunction with the step-through (Figure 19 and Figure 20) can be used to get over a low wall or similar obstacle. Find a suitable stable surface that is just above waist height. Place your palms flat on the surface, shoulder-width apart. Simultaneously jump into position and push down into your palms. Your shoulders should be depressed (as in the active hang) and directly over your hands. Your elbows should be fully extended. Your toes should be pushing into the wall and you should maintain tension throughout your body (Figure 34). Work on increasing the frequency and duration of the wall support hold in a similar way to the bar hang protocol.

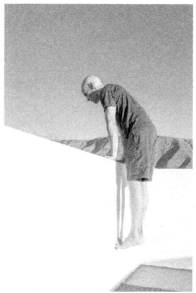

Figure 34: Wall support

CRAWLING

You were once well versed at crawling. It was a skill you taught yourself through trial and error as a baby, but is now probably long-forgotten. Crawling refers to low-to-the-ground quadrupedal movements, and there are many different types. We will focus on the basic bear and crab crawls. Crawling becomes a useful skill when you spend more time sitting on the ground, or in a full squat, rather than sitting on the couch (you have already adopted this habit, right?). Let's say you are sat down on your floor at home and want to get a magazine from the coffee table that is only a few feet away, it makes sense to crawl there. It is also a useful skill for scrambling up and down steep, loose terrain. It is also good for reinforcing cross-limb movement patterns and for improving mobility, strength and conditioning. Crawling can be tough at first (it requires: coordination, wrist strength and shoulder, spine and pelvis stability) so we will begin with some precursor exercises.

Stabilizing your shoulders

Begin on all fours with your knees directly underneath your hips, your arms straight and your wrists directly underneath your shoulders. To protect your wrists, distribute most of the load across your fingertips rather than on the heels of your hands (imagine gripping the ground). Depress your shoulder blades (move them down your back) and avoid letting your shoulders sag and collapse. Externally rotate your arms by attempting to corkscrew your hands outwards (note: your hands should not move, but your elbow pits should be facing forward). The corkscrew tension stabilizes your shoulder joints. Maintaining stable shoulders is important during crawling as well as other exercises such as the push-up.

Push-up

From the all-fours position described above, maintain upper body tension and step your legs back into the top position of the push-up (Figure 35).

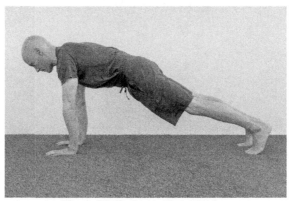

Figure 35: Push-up: Top position

Flex your elbows and slowly lower your chest to the ground, inhaling as you do so. Your upper arms should be near your sides with your elbows pointing backwards (Figure 36). Avoid the popular flared-elbows style as this puts unnecessary stress on the shoulder joints. Exhale while slowly pushing back up to the start position.

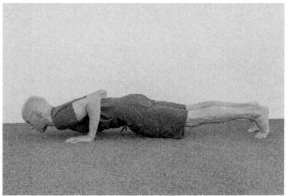

Figure 36: Push-up: Bottom position

The push-up is quite a tough exercise and you may find that you do not have the requisite strength to perform it from the get-go. If this is the case, you should opt for the regression version. With the push-up regression exercise you use regular push-up form but reduce the resistance by placing your hands on a raised stable surface (Figure 37). Initially the surface may need to be relatively high, such as a wall at waist height. Then as you improve you can use progressively lower surfaces. Before attempting the push-up regression exercise ensure the surface is safe and stable and can bear your body weight.

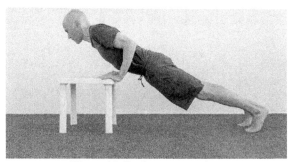
Figure 37: Push-up regression

Head nods in sphinx
Adopt the sphinx posture (Figure 38). Leading with your eyes, look upwards as far as you can and extend your neck. Leading with eyes, look downwards and flex your neck so your chin gets as close as possible to your chest. Repeat this nodding action whilst keeping your shoulders depressed.

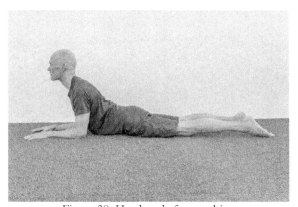
Figure 38: Head nods from sphinx

Static limb raises

Get in a crawling position with your hands, knees, and the tops of your feet in contact with the ground (six points of contact). Your wrists should be directly underneath your shoulders, and your knees directly underneath your hips. This is called the six-point bear crawl position. Keeping the rest of your body motionless, raise your left hand a few centimetres off the ground. Place it back on the ground. Now raise your right hand a few centimetres off the ground. Place it back on the ground. Raise your right knee and foot a few centimetres off the ground. Place them back on the ground and raise your left knee and foot a few centimetres off the ground. Place them back on the ground. Now reverse the direction. Once you have mastered this sequence you can progress to a contralateral pattern: raise your left hand and right knee and foot simultaneously, replace them and raise your right hand and left knee and foot simultaneously.

Six-point bear crawl

Crawling is an excellent exercise for developing strength and conditioning; it can be strenuous, yet very safe. We will start with the easier six-points-of-contact version.

From the bear crawl position, move your left knee forward and your left hand backwards so they meet, this is your "short side". Your right limbs are apart, this is your "long side". You are now in the start position (Figure 39). If you get out of synchrony during crawling, it is also a useful "reset" position.

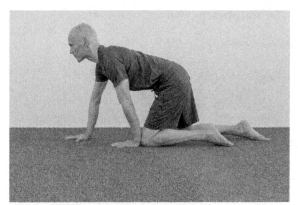

Figure 39: Six-point bear crawl: Start/reset position

From the start position, commence crawling by simultaneously stepping forward with your left hand and right knee (Figure 40). Then take a step with the opposite limbs. This cross-limb pattern is called a contralateral movement. As you crawl keep your head up and your gaze to the front (similar to head position in the sphinx exercise).

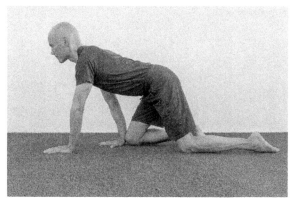

Figure 40: Six-point bear crawl: Contralateral step

When you first attempt crawling you may notice that your torso is twisting, be mindful and try to eliminate this; have a partner place a tennis ball on the small of your back and try and crawl without it falling off. You may also find that you drift into an ipsilateral pattern (both limbs on the same side of the body move together), if so stop, adopt the reset position, and then commence in a contralateral pattern. Also, practice reversing the movement and crawling backwards. You will need to look back over the shoulder of your "short side" with each step (Figure 41).

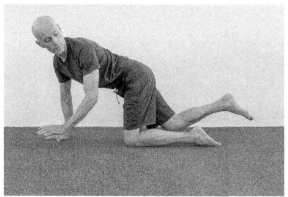

Figure 41: Six-point bear crawl: Contralateral step backwards

Four-point bear crawl

In essence this is the same movement as the previous crawl, only now you curl your toes under and raise your knees a few centimetres off the ground (Figure 42).

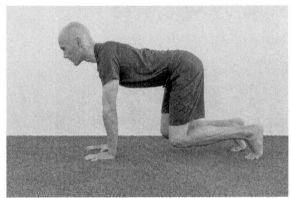

Figure 42: Four-point bear crawl position

This reduces your support base to four points of contact (hands and feet) and makes the exercise a lot tougher. Avoid the temptation to raise your knees higher off the ground as this makes the movement easier. Practice crawling forwards (Figure 43) and backwards (Figure 44).

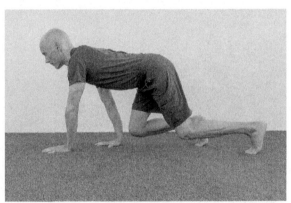

Figure 43: Four-point bear crawl: Contralateral step

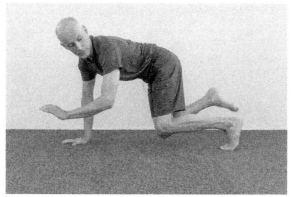

Figure 44: Four-point bear crawl: Contralateral step backwards

If four-point bear crawling is too much of a challenge, just holding the static position is an excellent way to develop the strength and conditioning needed for the dynamic version. You can also perform the static limb raise sequence to develop your fitness (in a similar fashion to that described earlier for the six-point bear crawl position).

Crab crawl

Sit down with your knees bent and your feet on the ground. Support yourself from behind with your hands. Stabilize your shoulders by depressing and retracting your shoulder blades. Raise your backside a few centimetres off the ground. This is the crab crawl position (Figure 45).

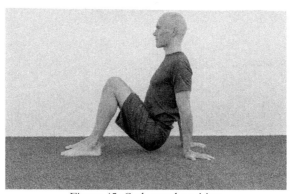

Figure 45: Crab crawl position

Begin with your left hand and left foot relatively close (short side) and your right hand and right leg somewhat apart (long side). Your hands should be in a comfortable position (Figure 46).

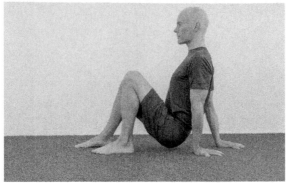

Figure 46: Crab crawl: Start/reset position

Crawl forward in a contralateral pattern, simultaneously stepping forward with your left foot and right hand (Figure 47).

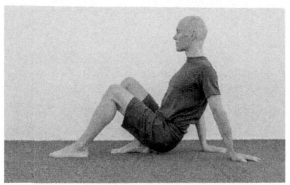

Figure 47: Crab crawl: Contralateral step

Repeat with your right foot and left hand. Throughout the movement maintain stability in your shoulder girdle. Practice crawling forwards and backwards.

Step-through transition
The step-through is a movement pattern that can be used as a transition between bear crawling and crab crawling. From a static crab position, lift your right hand and left foot off the ground (Figure 48).

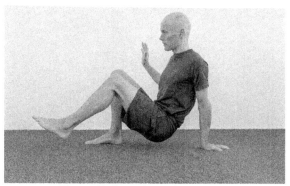

Figure 48: Step-through transition

Rotate using the weight of your body, so that your left leg goes underneath you (Figure 49). Place your right hand and left foot on the ground in the bear crawl position (Figure 50).

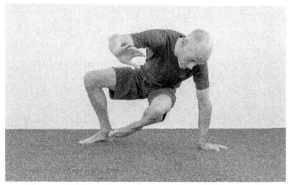

Figure 49: Step-through transition (underswitch)

51

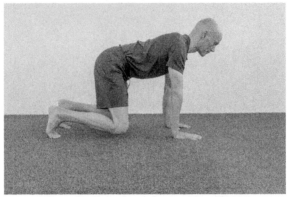

Figure 50: Step-through transition (finish)

Reverse the movement back into the crab position. Practice the transition in the opposite direction: lift your left hand and right foot off the ground, rotate so that your right leg goes underneath you, place your left hand and right foot on the ground in the bear crawl position.

SAFETY, SCALING AND COACHING

As mentioned previously, good form is paramount. It is therefore important to be able to scale your movements to suit your current capacity. By this I mean the movement task you are aiming to learn should be simple and not too physically demanding. This is a safe way to learn a movement. Trying to learn a skill when fatigued is not a good idea. Once you have mastered the simple version of the movement you can then challenge yourself with a slightly more complex or physically demanding version. This approach will safely ensure continual growth. However, there is no substitute for a good quality coach when learning new movements. I therefore recommend you seek the advice of a professional movement coach: it is the safest and most efficient way to progress.

Slowly and carefully work your way through the movements highlighted in this chapter to determine whether you can perform them safely, correctly and with control. Continue working through them until you can perform them efficiently. This in itself will be a rewarding and challenging practice. You can then begin to link several movements in sequence and develop your transition skills. Do not be overly concerned with reps and sets, instead pay attention to correct form. Begin your practice with easy versions of the movements in order to warm-up and get yourself prepared. Once you are fully warmed-up, you can increase the intensity to a moderate level. Remember to breathe through your nose and avoid holding your breath. If you notice your form waning due to fatigue, terminate the session and come back to it at a later time.

You will notice that once you become proficient at the above movements you can start using them in everyday tasks. As more movement options become available to you, your movement practice becomes integrated into your everyday life and your daily activities then become your movement practice, which is our end goal.

MOVEMENT RIDDLES

As we have seen, being sedentary, or following a gym-based training regime, can lead to movement illiteracy and the inability to move properly. In these situations we chunk body parts together and forget how to move in a nuanced way. The reduced stimuli cause our neural pathways to atrophy and we develop movement amnesia.

By way of illustration, consider a child who is monkeying around and playing on a climbing frame. The parent challenges the child to perform a chin-up. The child tries, but fails. The parent coaches the child and then one day following considerable practice the child performs a chin-up. The parent then encourages the child to perform several repetitions, then sets of repetitions. On the surface this may seem like a success, but it is not. The child has gone from engaging in creative, problem solving, fun movements to focusing on a single, specific movement pattern. The child has also learned that quantity (reps and sets) is prized over the quality of movement.

Movement riddles are the antithesis of repetitive movement. Consider for a moment how well learned your own movement patterns are. Cross your arms. Now repeat, only this time in the mirror image. Notice how strange it feels and how you have to think about it. Rather than learn a movement, repeat it, then load it for reps and sets, movement riddles set you a challenge and once you have solved it, you move on to the next one. This approach continually keeps you learning, keeps your movements creative, reduces chronic wear and tear, and avoids movement amnesia. It is also fun and keeps you young!

Worked example: Bouldering

Bouldering is a great example of a movement riddle. Bouldering is a subset of climbing and is performed without ropes. This may sound foolhardy, but typical bouldering problems only require a handful of moves and finish relatively low to the ground. When a problem is completed the boulderer will down-climb or jump the short distance to the ground. Typically, a portable crash mat is used to provide a safer landing. Certain handholds and footholds are allowed depending upon the difficulty of the problem, and most bouldering problems contain a crux move which is the main challenge of the problem. For a particular venue, guidebooks and topos are available which provide a range of problems of varying grades.

The challenge for the boulderer is to solve the problem, which in essence is a movement riddle. Once a problem is solved (a process that often takes several attempts) the boulderer moves on to tackle another one. Very rarely do boulderers continually repeat a problem they have previously solved. They may move on to another of a similar grade or push their abilities on a tougher one. In order to improve, boulderers not only have to improve their strength and mobility, but they also have to develop an increased body awareness and movement literacy. This draw to keep pushing their grade provides the motivation to develop their fitness.

Over recent years indoor climbing gyms and bouldering centres have become increasingly popular. This has meant that bouldering can be accessed with relative ease by the general public. Here routes are graded and colour coded accordingly. Every month or so a professional problem-setter will be tasked with setting new problems which ensures an endless supply of movement riddles.

It is worth giving bouldering a try if you have never done it before. You never know, it might be one of those activities that resonates with you. In the beginning it is advisable to seek out a skilled coach to show you the basic techniques and highlight the relevant health and safety procedures. However, if you find bouldering is not for you, no problem, at least you have tried to move your body differently.

WAY LEADS ONTO WAY

Nearly three decades ago when I first became interested in bouldering it was clear that in order to improve I needed to improve my hip mobility. I focused on developing this area of my fitness, mainly through yoga, and my bouldering improved. I also had an immediate connection with yoga and have practised it daily ever since. Which in turn has lead me on to many other movement practices.

If you cannot swim, take lessons. Try different martial arts classes. Try different sports. Tend your garden, or help your neighbours do theirs. Try whatever activity you like. You do not have to do all of the activities all of the time: just get proficient and then move on, returning on occasion to avoid developing any movement blind spots. Get creative. Get moving!

Play

There is an important philosophical difference between movement practice and the prevalent gym and studio-based training. You are human and you are greater than the sum of your fitness components: you are not just muscle tissue that needs to get bigger or cardiac tissue that needs to beat faster. You need to play! Yet play for adults is readily dismissed. Play is a great learning experience, it nurtures curiosity, creativity, innovation and critical thinking. Play also enables us to develop intellectually, emotionally and behaviourally. And play keeps ageing at bay.

In an ideal world you would get all of your movement nutrition from your daily living and play. This is the standard you should strive for. However, in the real world this is probably not feasible. No worries. Get into the habit of performing a mental movement audit and appraise your weekly movement engagement. If you have not touched the ground for a few days, crawl around for a bit. If you feel tight in your hips attend a yoga class or include a variety of sitting positions into your day and play with transitioning from one to another. If it has been a while since you last climbed something, go bouldering. You get the idea.

CHAPTER SEVEN:
RESISTANCE EXERCISE

We will use resistance exercise solely as a tool to address the shortfall between your current physical activity level and the ideal physical activity profile highlighted in Figure 4, Chapter Four. As you will recall, your ideal activity profile should include a maximum of two resistance exercise sessions per week. In this chapter we will explore what these resistance exercises are and how you should integrate them into your weekly activity profile.

We need resistance exercise to enhance our health and fitness. However, exercise is a stress and too much stress (distress) can be harmful to health. Therefore the goal for our resistance exercise sessions is to apply the optimal amount of stress (eustress) to promote adaptation and elicit the maximum benefits, and no more. If you do any more than the minimum effective load, you are merely exercising for exercising's sake and subjecting yourself to undue distress and hastening the ageing process, which is not something we want to do. Resistance exercise is simply a tool, the purpose of which is to develop your health and fitness and prepare you for your daily living and the things you want to do in your recreation time.

MOVEMENT PATTERNS
In the previous chapter we noted that humans are generalist movers capable of a considerable range of movement patterns. For the purpose of practicality we can categorize these movements into five main areas: i) squat, ii) hinge, iii) vertical push and pull, iv) horizontal push and pull, and v) rotation and anti-rotation. These categories will be the focus of the resistance exercises.

Squat

The squat movement pattern involves maximum hip and knee flexion. In the bottom position your feet should be hip-width apart, parallel and your heels on the ground. Your centre of mass should be positioned over your forefeet (Figure 51).

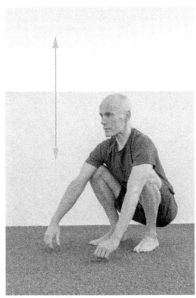

Figure 51: Squat movement pattern

Hinge

The hinge movement pattern involves hip flexion. Your lower legs should be vertical and your knees should be slightly flexed (Figure 52). With stable legs and a neutral spine, flex at the hips lowering your torso until your hands are level with your knees when your arms are straight (note: you do not support your hands on your knees). Your body weight should be predominantly supported by your hamstrings (back of thighs) and your gluteal (backside) muscles. If your hamstrings are tight and you cannot achieve this range of motion, don't worry; it is something to aim for. Avoid compensating by rounding your back to achieve the desired range.

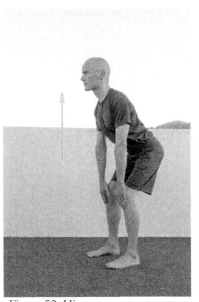

Figure 52: Hinge movement pattern

Vertical push and pull

A vertical push requires the arms to push against an overhead resistance. A vertical pull requires the arms to pull against an overhead resistance (Figure 53). This should be performed with the elbows pointing forward, rather than flared out to the sides.

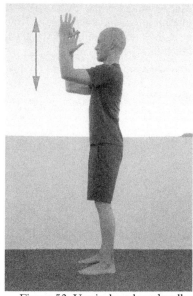

Figure 53: Vertical push and pull

Horizontal push and pull

A horizontal push requires the arms to push against a resistance in front of the body. A horizontal pull requires the arms to pull against a resistance in front of the body (Figure 54). This should be performed with your arms close to your body rather than flared out to the sides.

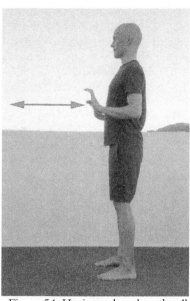

Figure 54: Horizontal push and pull

Rotation and anti-rotation

Rotation requires the torso to twist in opposition to a resistance. Anti-rotation requires the torso to remain static against a rotational resistance (Figure 55).

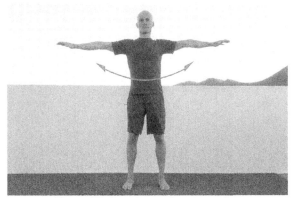

Figure 55: Rotation and anti-rotation

TIME UNDER TENSION

The widely adopted training modality based around multiple sets and reps in order to develop muscular strength and size certainly works. The evidence is plain for us to see in any weight room anywhere in the world. However, it is not the most efficient way to achieve the desired results, or the best way to age successfully. Furthermore, it can often lead to the 'more is better' mindset and proselytize exercising for exercising's sake. This is a time consuming approach and it adds unnecessary exercise distress. To avoid this trap and to optimize your efforts you need only be concerned with: i) correct form, ii) exercise intensity, and iii) time under tension. These are key determinants for developing muscular strength and muscle mass, both of which are linked to successful ageing.

  We will be using exercise protocols based on isometric (static) contractions and slow repetitions. A benefit of these protocols is there is no (or minimal) momentum or acceleration involved thus reducing the likelihood of injury (compared with free weight exercises). This makes these modes of resistance exercise safe. In addition, they require minimal equipment and can be performed pretty much anywhere.

IMPORTANT

For healthy people, isometric exercises are very safe. However, if you suffer from cardiovascular disease and/ or hypertension (high blood pressure) isometric exercises may be contraindicated and potentially cause harm. It is therefore imperative that you heed the advice in the DISCLAIMER at the beginning of this book, and before changing your lifestyle you should seek medical advice from your General Practitioner/ Physician regarding your specific circumstances.

Each resistance exercise session will comprise: a warm-up, seven resistance exercises, and a cool-down.

WARM-UP
Before engaging in the resistance exercise sessions you should perform a warm-up to prepare your body for the exercises. There are many options for your warm-up and to a large degree it will be determined by your condition on the day and where you are feeling tight and stiff. If I have the time available I like to spend between 30 - 45 minutes warming-up, primarily because I enjoy it.

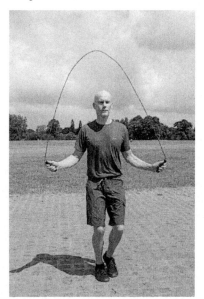

However, my default warm-up routine if I am pushed for time is five minutes of boxer-style skipping (Figure 56) followed by ten minutes of sun salutations (Figures 57 to 68). I recommend doing no less than this. (If you have the time you can extend your mobility phase by incorporating some of the movements described in Chapter Six).

The intensity of your skipping should be determined by your nasal breathing. Focus on your breath and bring your mind to the present moment. When you are ready, move onto the sun salutations.

Figure 56: Skipping

Sun salutations
We will borrow from yoga here. The sun salutation (surya namaskara) sequence is an excellent way to move your body in preparation for the resistance exercises. It is a short routine linking twelve postures (asanas). I particularly like this sequence as it encourages you to flow gracefully from one asana to the next in synchrony with your breath.

Posture 1: Sunrise (Pranamasana)

Breathing: Nasal exhale

Stand upright, gazing forward with the palms of your hands together in front of your chest (Figure 57). There should be a slight pressure between your hands. Fully exhale before moving to the next asana.

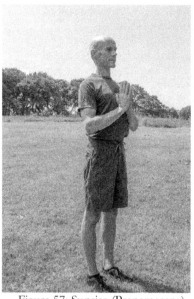

Figure 57: Sunrise (Pranamasana)

Posture 2: Raised arms (Hasta uttanasana)

Breathing: Nasal inhale

During the inhale raise your arms above your head and stretch high (Figure 58). There should be a slight back bend here, but take care not to hyperextend. Stay within your comfort zone.

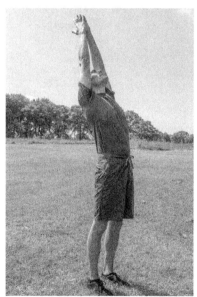

Figure 58: Raised arms (Hasta uttanasana)

Posture 3: Forward bend (Padahastasana)

Breathing: Nasal exhale

During the exhale, bend forward at the hips and lower your hands to the ground, or as far as is comfortable (Figure 59). Your knees should bend slightly.

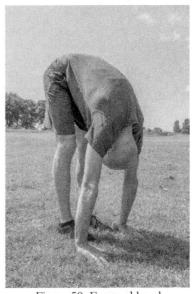

Figure 59: Forward bend (Padahastasana)

Posture 4: Equestrian (Ashva Sanchalanasana)

Breathing: Nasal inhale

During the inhale, move your right foot backwards and let your right knee touch the ground, whilst simultaneously bending your left knee (Figure 60). Your fingers should be touching the ground. As you finish your inhale expand your chest. (Note: on the next complete sequence switch legs).

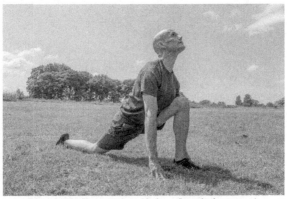

Figure 60: Equestrian (Ashva Sanchalanasana)

Posture 5: Downward- facing dog (Adho mukha svanasana)

Breathing: Nasal exhale

During the exhale, move your left foot inline with your right foot whilst raising your hips. Aim to get your arms and legs as straight as possible. Your head should be between your arms (Figure 61).

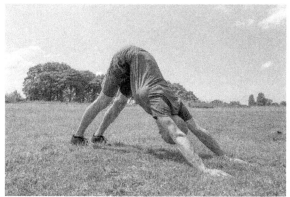

Figure 61: Downward- facing dog (Adho mukha svanasana)

Posture 6: Eight limbs (Astangasana)

Breathing: momentary pause

During this brief transitional posture you should momentarily suspend your breathing. Lower yourself down so that you have eight parts of your body touching the ground: two hands, two feet, two knees, chest and chin (Figure 62).

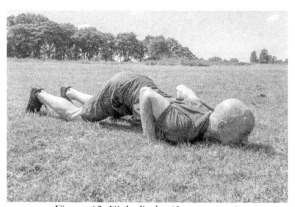

Figure 62: Eight limbs (Astangasana)

Posture 7: Cobra (Bhujangasana)
Breathing: Nasal inhale
During the inhale use your back muscles to extend your spine, move your hips to the ground and look upwards (Figure 63). Avoid over reliance on your arms.

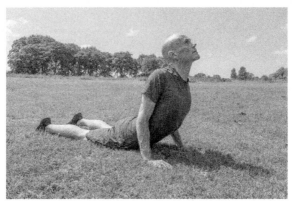
Figure 63: Cobra (Bhujangasana)

Posture 8: Downward- facing dog (Adho mukha svanasana)
Breathing: Nasal exhale
During the exhale raise your hips upwards. Aim to get your arms and legs as straight as possible. Your head should be between your arms (Figure 64).

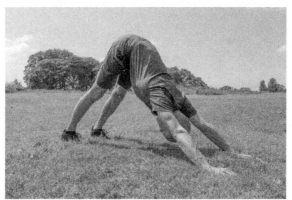
Figure 64: Downward- facing dog (Adho mukha svanasana)

Posture 9: Equestrian (Ashva Sanchalanasana)
Breathing: Nasal inhale
During the inhale, bring your right foot forward in line with your hands and let your left knee touch the ground. Your fingers should be touching the ground

(Figure 65). As you finish your inhale expand your chest. (Note: on the next complete sequence switch legs).

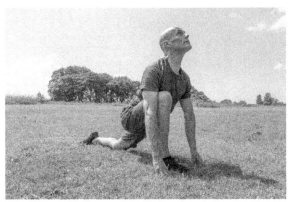
Figure 65: Equestrian (Ashva Sanchalanasana)

Posture 10: Forward bend (Padahastasana)
Breathing: Nasal exhale
During the exhale, move your left foot next to your right foot and move into a forward bend. Your knees should bend slightly (Figure 66).

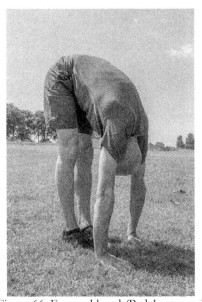
Figure 66: Forward bend (Padahastasana)

Posture 11: Raised arms (Hasta uttanasana)

Breathing: Nasal inhale

During the inhale stand up and stretch high (Figure 67). There should be a slight back bend here, but take care not to hyperextend. Stay within your comfort zone.

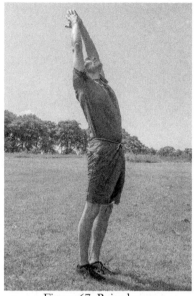

Figure 67: Raised arms (Hasta uttanasana)

Posture 12: Sunset (Pranamasana)

Breathing: Nasal exhale

As you exhale, bring the arms back down in front of the chest as you return to the beginning posture (Figure 68).

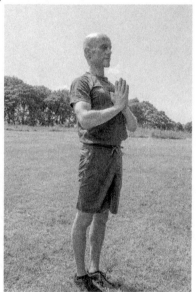

Figure 68: Sunset (Pranamasana)

Perform the above sequence for 10 minutes and as you warm up move further into the postures so that you feel a comfortable stretch. Only begin the resistance exercises when you are ready.

COOL-DOWN
To facilitate recovery after the resistance exercise sessions, keep yourself moving at a low intensity by walking around for a few minutes. Then slowly perform a few more sequences of the sun salutations. If you wish, you can take your time and hold the stretches for several breaths (up to 30 seconds).

TYPES OF MUSCULAR CONTRACTION
There are three main classifications of muscle action: concentric, eccentric and isometric. A concentric muscle contraction occurs when the tension in the muscle overcomes the resistance and the muscle shortens, such as lifting a load. Eccentric muscle contraction involves the muscle lengthening under tension, such as lowering a load. Isometric muscle contraction occurs when tension is generated but the muscle does not change length, such as contracting against an immovable object, or holding a load.

For the resistance exercises detailed in this chapter (indeed all of the activities in this book) it is important to avoid the temptation to hold your breath or perform the Valsalva manoeuvre. The Valsalva manoeuvre involves attempting to forcefully exhale against a closed airway, it sounds like a grunt, and unfortunately it is the soundtrack of most gyms. The reason to avoid these practices is they are associated with increasing intrathoracic pressure, which in turn causes increases in systolic and diastolic blood pressure. To further reduce unnecessary elevations in blood pressure whilst exercising, avoid the temptation to contract those muscles not involved in the exercise, such as when you over-grip, squirm or grimace. Instead, remain calm, only create tension in the required muscles, keep a relaxed face and breathe through your nose. Use your breathing as a guide. Once each exercise is completed walk around and give your aerobic system time to allow you to fully recover before moving onto the next one.

RESISTANCE EXERCISES: ISOMETRICS
Isometrics are not new, they have been part of physical culture since time immemorial. The strongmen of the late 1800s and early 1900s such as Eugen Sandow, Alexander Zass and Charles Atlas popularized isometric exercise and brought it to the general public's conscious. Since then isometric exercise has come in and out of vogue. More recently, trainers such as Ken Hutchins and Drew Baye have developed isometric exercise protocols with evidence-based demonstrable health and fitness benefits.

During the last 35 years I have integrated isometrics into my own strength exercise practice in one form or another to great effect. However, it was only relatively recently while training with American fitness coach Steve Maxwell that I learned of the benefits to be gained from a strength session comprised entirely of isometric exercises. They are now a key part of my strength development. There are many different isometric exercises and protocols available, but those detailed in this chapter are the ones that I have found most beneficial to health and can be effectively integrated into the ideal weekly physical activity profile (Figure 4, Chapter Four).

Detailed below are two isometric resistance exercise protocols: the yielding isometric session and the overcoming isometric session. Each one is a stand-alone resistance exercise session that can be integrated into your ideal weekly physical activity profile (Figure 4, Chapter Four). Each protocol comprises seven exercises and each exercise is performed for 90 seconds, giving a cumulative 10 minutes 30 seconds under tension. You may be surprised by the short duration of the exercise sessions, however the time under tension is significant and it efficiently produces the desired results.

Equipment
You will need a basic timer and a suitable, sturdy strap. In the exercises described below I am using a heavy-duty furniture moving strap, I like this because it is wide and comfortable and has convenient loops at the ends. This type of strap is not a prerequisite; there are many equally suitable alternatives such as a heavy-duty tie-down/ towing strap (Figure 69), or even a martial arts belt. If your tie down strap has a cam-buckle it is possible to make a loop which can be used in conjunction with a dowel to make the exercises more comfortable (see the specific exercise descriptions later). When using the strap you may want to wrap the free ends around your hands to increase your grip.

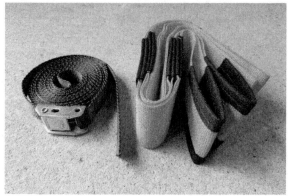

Figure 69: Tie-down strap (left) and furniture removal strap (right)

Yielding isometric session

Yielding isometric exercises require you to support a resistance; over time your muscles will tire and you will eventually yield to the load. For the majority of the exercises in this session the resistance will be your body weight. When using a structure for support, or to act as an anchor point for the strap, always check that it is safe and secure and can bear your body weight before performing the exercises.

Protocol

Perform the sequence of exercises once. Fully recover between each exercise. Complete the exercises in order and statically hold each one for 90 seconds. The concept is to apply a challenging resistance, one that will momentarily fatigue your working muscles at the end of 90 seconds. As a rule of thumb your starting intensity should be at a moderate level (equivalent to 30-40% of what you predict your maximal effort to be) and you should maintain this same level of tension for the duration of the exercise. This is a safe protocol because, despite the last part of the 90 seconds becoming fatiguing and your perceived exertion rising, the tension in your muscles is still only moderate (compared to your predicted maximum).

Due to the nature of biomechanics, there are difficult and easy ranges of motion for each exercise. For example, in the squat exercise the top third of the range of motion is relatively easy compared to the middle or bottom thirds. If you are new to exercise, the top third may provide a sufficient challenge and you should start here. Whereas if you require more resistance, you will find it in the middle third. For each exercise find the part of the range of motion that initially equates to a moderate effort and hold it. As your strength improves, in subsequent sessions you can progress the starting range of motion accordingly.

Gauging the starting intensity (range of motion or tension) is not an exact science and it may take a few sessions to get it dialled. So in the beginning err on the side of caution and opt for a reduced initial intensity, which you can then fine-tune in future sessions.

Remember to maintain your nasal breathing throughout the exercises and avoid any temptation to hold your breath. Focus on creating tension only in those muscles being used and relax those not in use.

Squat

Hold an isometric squat position (Figure 70). Cross your arms and place your hands on opposite shoulders. Keep your shins parallel to each other and avoid allowing your knees to collapse inwards. Keep your spine neutral, look ahead and do your best to keep your torso as upright as possible. Follow the 90 second moderate-intensity isometric protocol. Fully recover before progressing onto the next exercise.

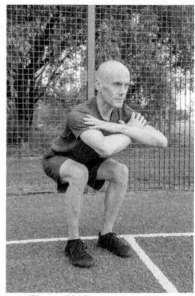

Figure 70: Isometric squat

Hinge

Hold an isometric hinge position (Figure 71). Cross your arms and place your hands on opposite shoulders. Your hips should be flexed and your knees should have a slight bend. Your lower legs should be vertical with the load being supported predominantly by your hamstrings (back of thighs) and your gluteal (backside) muscles. You may need to make micro adjustments until you feel these muscles working. It is important that you make this mind-muscle link and can engage these muscles before progressing and adding extra resistance. Follow the 90 second moderate-intensity isometric protocol. Fully recover before progressing onto the next exercise.

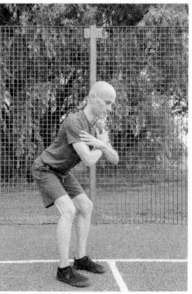

Figure 71: Isometric hinge

To reduce the loading of the isometric hinge, place your hands on your hips. To increase the resistance, you can place your hands behind your head, or to increase it further raise your arms overhead (known as chair pose, Figure 72).

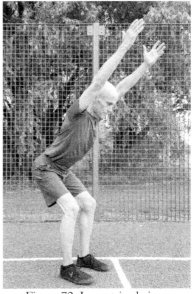

Figure 72: Isometric chair (progression)

Vertical push

For the vertical push you will need to find a moderate load that you can support for 90 seconds (in Figure 73 I am using water bottles). Your upper arms should be horizontal and in front of you, with your forearms vertical. Follow the 90 second moderate-intensity isometric protocol. Fully recover before progressing onto the next exercise.

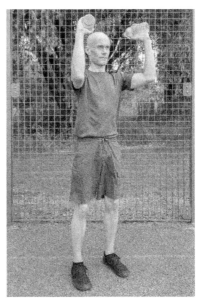

Figure 73: Isometric vertical push with water bottles

Vertical pull

Depending upon what is available to you, there are a couple of options for the vertical pull. Place your strap over a sturdy overhead structure and take hold of either end. Adopt the position shown in Figure 74: your torso should be vertical, your upper arms should be horizontal and your elbows should be pointing forwards and bent at 90 degrees. Hold the position by creating tension by "pulling with your elbows" rather than your biceps. You can modulate the resistance applied to your upper body by altering the contribution from your legs. Follow the 90 second moderate-intensity isometric protocol. Fully recover before progressing onto the next exercise.

Alternatively you can use a horizontal bar at a suitable height (Figure 75).

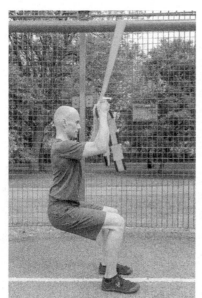 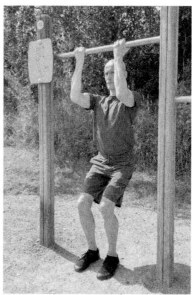

Figure 74: Isometric vertical pull with strap | Figure 75: Isometric vertical pull on low bar

Horizontal push

Adopt the isometric elevated push-up position (Figure 76). Stand approximately a stride length away from a stable elevated surface, place your hands on the surface and lean until your elbows are bent at 90 degrees and close to your sides. Your ankles, knees, hips and shoulders should be in a straight line. To achieve a moderate starting intensity, the surface may need to be relatively high, such as a wall at waist height. Follow the 90 second moderate-intensity isometric protocol. Fully recover before progressing onto the next exercise.

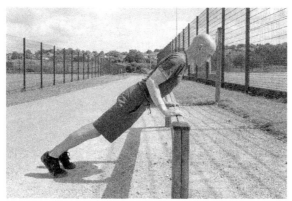

Figure 76: Isometric elevated push-up

As your fitness improves, use progressively lower surfaces until you can perform the isometric push-up on the ground as shown in Figure 77 (note: the starting intensity should only be moderate).

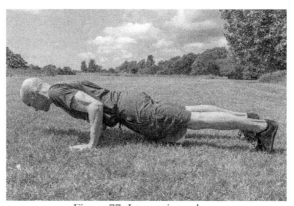

Figure 77: Isometric push-up

Horizontal pull

Stand facing a sturdy vertical post or pole. Securely place the strap around the post and ensure it will not slip. Grip the ends of the strap and lean back so that you are in the position shown in Figure 78. There should be a straight line through your ankles, knees, hips and shoulders. Your elbows should be by your sides and bent at 90 degrees. Hold the position by creating tension by "pulling with your elbows" rather than your biceps. You can increase the load by increasing the length of the strap.

If you are extremely fit and this provides less than a moderate starting intensity, you can increase the resistance further by adopting the position in Figure 79.

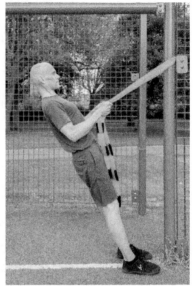

Figure 78: Isometric horizontal pull with strap

Wrap the strap around a sturdy horizontal bar. Sit underneath the bar and grasp the ends of the straps and pull yourself into position. There should be a horizontal line through your knees, hips, shoulders and head. Your elbows should be by your sides and bent at 90 degrees. Hold the position by creating tension by "pulling with your elbows" rather than your arms. Follow the 90 second moderate-intensity isometric protocol. Fully recover before progressing onto the next exercise.

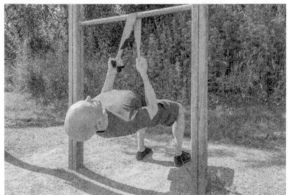

Figure 79: Isometric horizontal pull with strap (progression)

Anti-rotation

From a six-point crawling position, slowly raise and outstretch your right arm and your left leg. Maintain a steady body position for 45 seconds. Slowly return and repeat with opposite limbs for 45 seconds. This exercise is called the bird-dog (Figure 80).

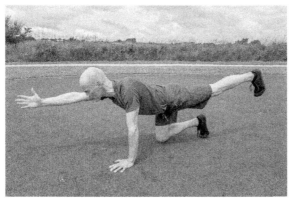

Figure 80: Foot, knee and hand bird-dog

Yielding isometric session exercise summary

Warm-up

Starting exercise intensity: moderate

1) Isometric squat (body weight)
2) Isometric hinge (progression: isometric chair)
3) Isometric vertical push with load (such as water bottles)
4) Isometric vertical pull with strap (or low bar)
5) Isometric elevated push-up (or isometric push-up)
6) Isometric horizontal pull with strap
7) Foot, knee and hand bird-dog

Cool-down

Overcoming isometric session

Overcoming isometrics is a term used to describe pushing against, or pulling on, an immovable object. For the majority of the exercises in this session the resistance will be provided by the strap. When using a structure for support, or to act as an anchor point for the strap, always check that it is safe and secure and can bear your body weight before performing the exercises.

Protocol

Perform the sequence of exercises once, making sure you fully recover between each exercise. Complete the exercises in order and statically hold each one for 90 seconds. The concept is to apply a challenging resistance, one that will momentarily fatigue your muscles at the end of 90 seconds. As a rule of thumb your starting effort should be at a moderate level (equivalent to 30-40% of your predicted maximal effort) and you should maintain this same level of tension for the duration of the exercise.

To prevent injury, it is important that you avoid snatching or yanking against the strap. Instead, smoothly take up the strain at the start, and then at the end of the exercise gently ease off the tension and relax. Remember to maintain your nasal breathing throughout the exercises and avoid any temptation to hold your breath. Focus on creating tension only in those muscles being used and relax those not in use.

Squat

This exercise is going to be the same as the previous yielding isometric squat. However, if you are extremely fit and the yielding isometric squat provides less than a moderate starting intensity, you can increase the resistance by using a hybrid of yielding and overcoming isometrics. If this is the case, the following hybrid isometric squat exercise can be used instead. Put the strap comfortably across the back of your hips and cross it at the front (Figures 81 and 82). Ensure that the strap is on your hips and not on your lower back.

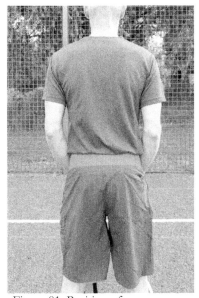

Figure 81: Position of strap across the hips

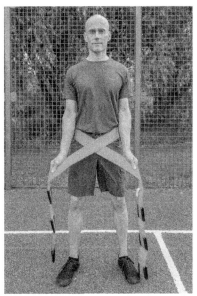

Figure 82: Strap crossed in front of the body

Step onto the ends of the strap with both feet and adjust it so that you are in the desired range (Figure 83). Cross your arms and place your hands on opposite shoulders. Keep your shins parallel to each other and avoid allowing your knees to collapse inwards. Keep your spine neutral, look ahead and do you best to keep your torso as upright as possible. Slowly take up the strain by pushing into the strap and follow the 90 second moderate-intensity isometric protocol. Fully recover before progressing onto the next exercise.

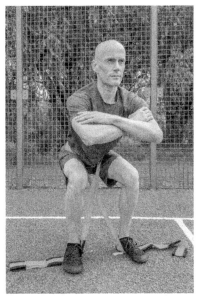

Figure 83: Isometric squat against strap

Getting this configuration right can be a bit difficult at first, but after a few attempts you will have it sorted. If you are using a strap without loops you may want to wrap the strap around your feet to prevent it from slipping. You will note that you can apply the resistance without your spine being loaded.

Hinge

Stand on the strap with your heels and grip the free ends so that your hands are approximately level with your knees (Figure 84). To maintain your grip on the strap you may need to wrap it around your hands. Sit back into the hinge posture, ensuring your lower legs are vertical and your back is not rounded. Your knees should be slightly flexed. Your glutes and hamstrings should be the predominant working muscles, not your lower back or quadriceps (front thighs). Slowly take up the strain by pulling on the strap and follow the 90 second moderate-intensity isometric protocol. Fully recover before progressing onto the next exercise.

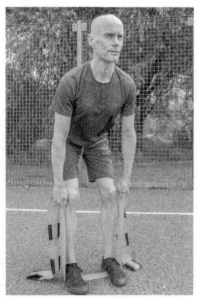 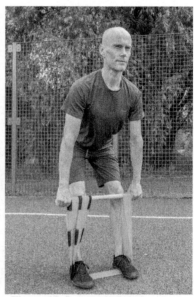

Figure 84: Isometric hinge against strap
Figure 85: Isometric hinge against strap with dowel

Alternatively, if you have a strap with loops, or a tie down with a cam buckle (so you can make one large loop) you can insert a sturdy dowel through the loops to give you a bar to hold on to (Figure 85). I find this makes the exercise more comfortable. Ensure the dowel is strong enough before using it. Fully recover before progressing onto the next exercise.

Vertical push

A sturdy horizontal bar at head height is ideal for this exercise. Grasp the bar with an overhand grip, elbows pointing forwards and bent at 90 degrees (Figure 86). Avoid the temptation to flare your elbows out wide (less than 45 degrees is ideal). Slowly take up the strain by pushing into the bar and follow the 90 second moderate-intensity isometric protocol. Fully recover before progressing onto the next exercise.

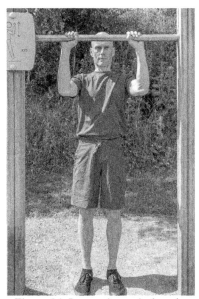

Figure 86: Isometric vertical push

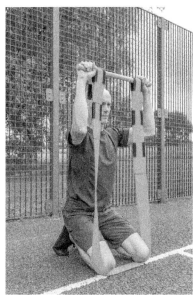

Figure 87: Isometric vertical push against strap with dowel

Alternatively, you can perform this exercise with the strap. Kneel on the middle of the strap and grip the ends so that your upper arms are horizontal and in front of you. Avoid the temptation to flare your elbows out wide (less than 45 degrees is ideal). Sit up tall, slowly take up the strain by pushing upwards into the strap. If your strap has loops you can also insert a sturdy dowel into the loops (Figure 87). I find this makes the exercise more comfortable. Ensure the dowel is strong enough before using it. Fully recover before progressing onto the next exercise.

Vertical pull

Securely anchor the ends of the strap from above by looping it over a suitable sturdy object. Grip the strap so that your upper arms are horizontal and your elbows are pointing forwards (Figure 88). Avoid the temptation to flare your elbows out wide (less than 45 degrees is ideal). Take up the strain by "pulling with your elbows" rather than your biceps and follow the 90 second moderate-intensity isometric protocol. Fully recover before progressing onto the next exercise.

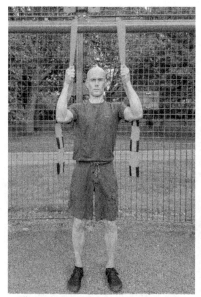 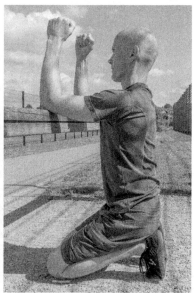

Figure 88: Isometric vertical pull against strap | Figure 89: Isometric vertical elbow pull

An alternative method is to place your elbows on a sturdy structure in front of you. Your upper arms should be horizontal and your elbows pointing forwards. Your torso should be upright (Figure 89). Slowly take up the strain by pushing down with your elbows (you may want to pad the surface) and follow the 90 second moderate-intensity isometric protocol. Fully recover before progressing onto the next exercise.

Horizontal push

Place the strap across your back and grip the ends so that your upper arms are vertical and next to your sides and your forearms are horizontal. Keeping your spine neutral, slowly take up the strain by pushing forward into the strap and follow the 90 second moderate-intensity isometric protocol (Figure 90). Fully recover before progressing onto the next exercise.

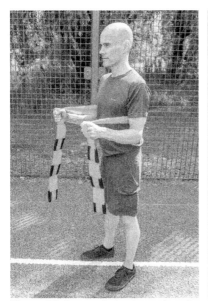 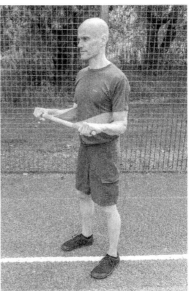

Figure 90: Isometric horizontal push against strap   Figure 91: Isometric horizontal push against strap with dowel

Alternatively, if your strap has loops you can insert a sturdy dowel into the loops (Figure 91). I find this makes the exercise more comfortable. Ensure the dowel is strong enough before using it. Fully recover before progressing onto the next exercise.

If you are extremely fit a further alternative is to use a hybrid of yielding and overcoming isometrics. Get into a low push-up position with the strap across your back and the free ends anchored under each hand (Figure 92). Adjust the length of the strap so that it is taut when your elbows are at 90 degrees. Keep your upper arms at your sides, take up the strain by pushing into the strap and follow the 90 second moderate-intensity isometric protocol. (Note: this is a tough exercise, and it is important to remember that the starting exercise intensity should only be moderate). Fully recover before progressing onto the next exercise.

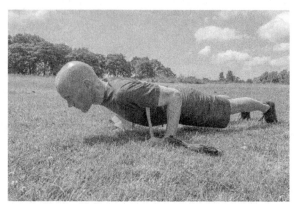

Figure 92: Isometric push-up against strap

Horizontal pull

Sit in an L-sit position, or staff posture, and loop the strap around your feet. Ensure your back is upright, bend your knees if it helps. Grip the ends of the strap so that your upper arms are vertical and next to your sides and your lower arms are horizontal (Figure 93). Take up the strain by pulling the strap "with your elbows" and follow the 90 second moderate-intensity protocol. Fully recover before progressing onto the next exercise.

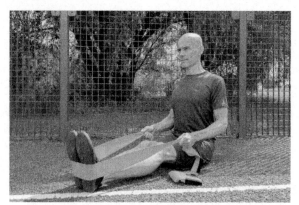

Figure 93: Isometric horizontal pull against strap

An alternative method is to lie supine on the ground. Your upper arms should be by your sides and your forearms vertical (Figure 94). Take up the strain by pushing into the ground with your elbows and follow the 90 second moderate-intensity protocol. Fully recover before progressing onto the next exercise.

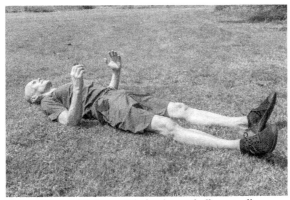
Figure 94: Isometric horizontal elbow pull

Anti-rotation
This is the same foot, knee and hand bird-dog exercise (Figure 80) as in the yielding isometric exercise session.

Overcoming isometric session exercise summary
Warm-up
Starting exercise intensity: moderate
1) Isometric squat (or against strap)
2) Isometric hinge against strap (or strap and dowel)
3) Isometric vertical push against bar (or strap/ and dowel)
4) Isometric vertical pull against strap (or vertical elbow pull)
5) Isometric horizontal push against strap (or strap and dowel, or push-up with strap)
6) Isometric horizontal pull against strap (or horizontal elbow pull)
7) Foot, knee and hand bird-dog
Cool-down

RESISTANCE EXERCISES: SLOW REPETITION
Performing slow repetitions is another way of safely developing muscle strength and hypertrophy. This series of exercises can be used as an alternative to the isometric series by way of providing variety.

Protocol
As the name suggests, you move through the range of motion slowly. The tempo should be four seconds to complete the shortening of the muscles (concentric phase) and four seconds to complete the lengthening of the muscles (eccentric phase). This is a safe form of exercise, however as with all forms of dynamic resistance training, the potential for harm is increased when there is a change in direction; with these exercises it is the transition between the

concentric and eccentric phases. You should aim to make these transitions as smooth and controlled as possible.

To maintain muscle tension throughout the exercises you should limit the range of motion to not include the easiest segment of the movement. If you are a beginner this may mean you avoid locking out your exercising limbs, whereas if you are very fit you may need to eliminate the easiest third. Choose a range of motion and intensity that enables you to continuously perform the repetitions until you reach momentary muscular fatigue after approximately 90 seconds without compromising correct form. As a rule of thumb the initial intensity should be moderate (equivalent to 30-40% of your predicted maximal effort). Remember to always remain calm and breathe through your nose. Do not hold your breath, do not grimace. Perform the sequence of exercises once, making sure you fully recover between each exercise.

Squat
Start facing a wall with your feet as close to the wall as possible and your arms out to the sides (Figure 95).

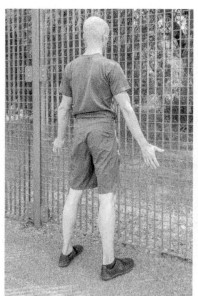 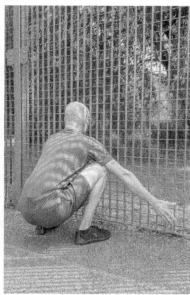

Figure 95: Slow-rep wall squat start   Figure 96: Slow rep wall squat
lowest point

Lower down over four seconds, hover momentarily (Figure 96), then slowly return to the top of your chosen range of motion and repeat. Make the transitions as smooth as possible. Fully recover before progressing onto the next exercise.

Depending upon the mobility at your hips, knees and ankles you may find that your range of motion is limited in this exercise. Don't be discouraged, work within your range without compromising form and in time your range of motion will increase.

Hinge

Stand facing away from a wall or sturdy post. Stand on your right leg and place the sole of your left foot against the wall. Adjust your position relative to the wall so that both of your knees are aligned. Put your hands on opposite shoulders (Figure 97).

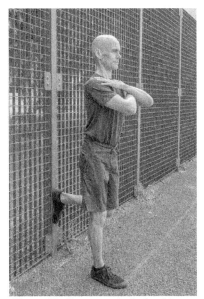
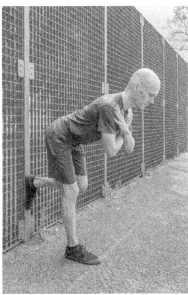

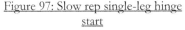

Figure 97: Slow rep single-leg hinge start

Figure 98: Slow rep single-leg hinge mid-point

Keep your back straight and slowly hinge forward at the hips for a count of four (Figure 98). The movement should only occur at your hips with your glutes and hamstrings being the predominant working muscles, not your lower back.

For a count of four return through your chosen range of motion and repeat. Throughout the movement aim to keep your knees aligned. Swap legs and repeat. Fully recover before progressing onto the next exercise.

Depending upon the mobility at your hips you may find that your range of motion is limited in this exercise. Don't be discouraged, work within your range without compromising form and in time your range of motion will increase.

To reduce the resistance, you can place your hands on your hips, or to increase the resistance you can place your hands behind your head.

Vertical push

From the starting position shown in Figure 99, slowly flex your elbows and lower your forehead towards your hands. Resist the temptation to flare your elbows out, instead keep them close to your body (Figure 100).

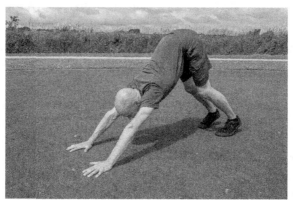

Figure 99: Dive-bomber push-up start

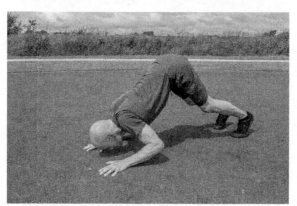

Figure 100: Dive-bomber push-up eccentric lower

Smoothly continue the dive-through by passing your chest between your hands, lowering your hips, straightening your arms and extending your back to look upwards (Figure 101). The movement from Figure 99 to Figure 101 should be performed smoothly over four seconds whilst inhaling through your nose. I find it helps to lead the movement with my eyes.

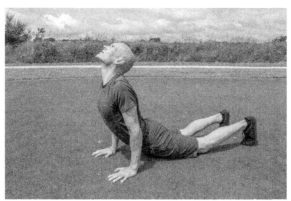

Figure 101: Dive-bomber push-up dive-through

At this juncture you have a couple of options to return to the start. The difficult option is reverse the process which requires a strong push from the position in Figure 100 back to that in Figure 99. This is called a Dive-bomber. During the return to the start position exhale through your nose.

A less strenuous move is from Figure 101, with straight arms, draw your pelvis up and back into the position in Figure 99. This is called a Dand push-up.

Even with the above adaptation, this can be a pretty tough exercise, so I have included a further regression below. From the position in Figure 99, keep your arms straight and lower your backside down into a bear squat (Figure 102).

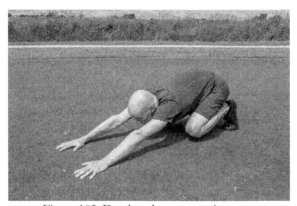

Figure 102: Dand push-up regression start

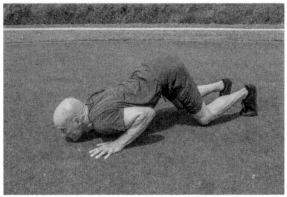

Figure 103: Dand push-up regression dive-through

This is the "new" start position. Leading with your eyes and keeping low, draw your chest between your hands (Figure 103) and smoothly continue the dive-through to finish position shown in Figure 101. Slowly return to the start position by sitting back into the bear squat. The easiest way to perform this regression is with your knees on the ground. You can make it more intense by hovering your knees a couple of centimetres off the ground. (Remember to select a version of this exercise that only requires a moderate starting intensity). Fully recover before progressing onto the next exercise.

Vertical pull

From an underhand grip hanging position (Figure 104), depress and retract your shoulder blades. For a count of four slowly draw your elbows down and backwards pulling yourself up until your chin is above the bar (Figure 105). This is called a chin-up. For a count of four, slowly lower yourself down stopping just shy of dead hanging and unweighting your muscles. Slowly pull yourself back up and repeat.

If this requires a greater than moderate starting intensity, you should use your legs for assistance. This can be achieved by placing your feet on a sturdy box, or by using a low bar (Figures 106 and 107). If you opt for assisted chin-ups modulate the assistance from your legs so that your starting intensity is moderate and you reach momentary muscular fatigue at around 90 seconds. Fully recover before progressing onto the next exercise.

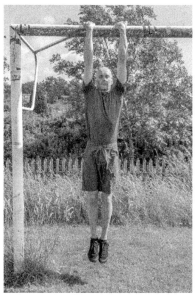
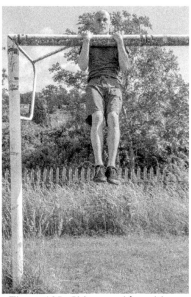

Figure 104: Chin-up start position Figure 105: Chin-up mid position

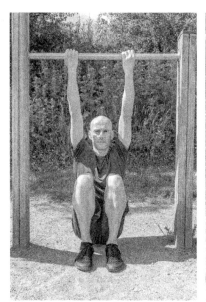
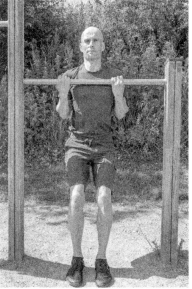

Figure 106: Assisted chin-up start position Figure 107: Assisted chin-up mid position

Horizontal push

From the top of the push-up position (Figure 108) slowly lower yourself for a count of four so your chest hovers about a fist-width above the ground (Figure 109).

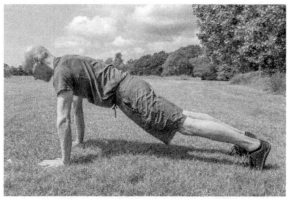

Figure 108: Push-up start position

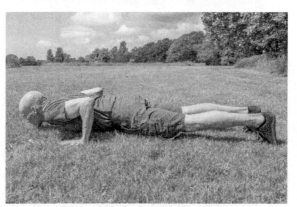

Figure 109: Push-up mid position

Slowly push up for a count of four. Then lower back down and repeat. Fully recover before progressing onto the next exercise. If this is too intense, you can reduce the intensity by placing your hands on an elevated stable surface (Figure 37: Push-up regression). To achieve a moderate starting intensity, the surface may need to be relatively high, such as a wall at waist height. As your fitness improves, you will be able to use progressively lower surfaces.

Horizontal pull

For this exercise you will need a suitable structure to hang your strap from. Ensure the strap is secure and will not slip. Grip the ends and lean back so that you are in the position shown in Figure 110. There should be a straight line through your ankles, knees, hips and shoulders.

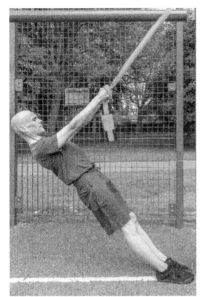 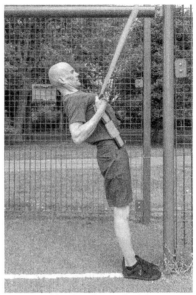

Figure 110: Horizontal pull with strap start   Figure 111: Horizontal with strap pull mid position

From a straight arm position, retract and depress your shoulders. For a count of four, pull your chest towards your hands using your back muscles (Figure 111). It helps to imagine pulling from your elbows rather than your hands.

For a count of four, slowly lower yourself back down through your desired range of motion and repeat. You can increase the load by increasing the length of the strap. Fully recover before progressing onto the next exercise.

Rotation and anti-rotation

This exercise is an advanced yielding isometric exercise. Adopt a six-point bear crawl position, and slowly raise and outstretch your right arm and your left leg (Figure 112). Maintain a steady body position and hold for 30 seconds. Whilst maintaining the outstretched position raise your right knee a couple of centimetres off the ground and hold for a further 15 seconds (Figure 113).

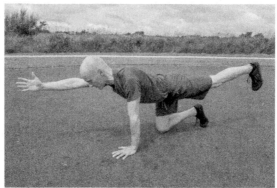

Figure 112: Foot, knee and hand bird-dog

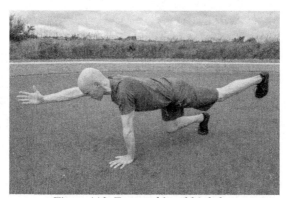

Figure 113: Foot and hand bird-dog

Immediately repeat on the other side. To progress this exercise, make the transition to the foot and hand bird-dog (Figure 113) earlier. To regress it, eliminate the knee lift and just perform the foot, knee and hand bird-dog (Figure 112).

Slow repetition exercise session summary
Warm-up
Starting exercise intensity: moderate
1) Wall squat
2) Single-leg hinge
3) Dive-bomber push-up (or Dand Push-up, or regression)
4) Assisted chin-up (or chin-up)
5) Elevated push-up (or push-up)
6) Horizontal pull with strap
7) Foot and hand bird-dog with transition (or foot, knee and hand bird-dog)
Cool-down

Integrating the resistance exercise sessions

The three resistance exercise protocols detailed above are stand-alone sessions. They form a pool for you to draw from when putting together your weekly resistance activities (Figure 4, Chapter Four). You can also create hybrid sessions by swapping exercises from the same movement pattern if you wish. For example, when doing the yielding isometric exercise session, you may find the isometric hinge too easy, in this instance you can swap in the isometric hinge against the strap. This latitude enables you to incorporate variety into your resistance exercise sessions, but crucially it gives you the option to choose those exercises from the specific movement patterns that allow you to begin the exercise at a moderate intensity. It is important to note that the exercise order within the resistance sessions must remain the same (squat, hinge, vertical push, vertical pull, horizontal push, horizontal pull, rotation/ anti-rotation).

As a guide, each week you should perform two resistance exercise sessions interspersed with a couple of recovery days. However, it is important to keep a watchful eye on how you are feeling and how much non-exercise resistance activity you are doing incidentally as you go about your week. If your week naturally involves some strength activities (such as heavy manual work) you should reduce the frequency of your resistance exercise sessions to just once in order to accommodate the extra stress. We also noted in Figure 4, Chapter Four that there should be an element of vigorous work in your weekly physical activity profile. This may come from participation in your chosen recreational activity. For example, if you roll on the mat in jujitsu, play squash or are involved in any fast-paced sport then this is probably enough. However, if your week has not called for any vigorous work, integrate some bouts of vigorous effort into your schedule, such as including a few short sprint intervals into your runs (ensure you are suitably warmed-up beforehand).

In summary, use the weekly physical activity pyramid (Figure 4, Chapter Four) as your general guide and tailor your resistance exercises and vigorous work to take up, or give you, slack.

CHAPTER EIGHT: PROVIDE WORTH

A common issue with regular health and fitness programmes is they are rooted in fear. The drivers of these programmes, such as, "I need to look good on holiday," or "I must lose weight," are pressuring and have an implied perilous consequence if they are not achieved. Sadly, this approach leaches intrinsic enjoyment from the process. Once (or should I say "if"?) the goal is achieved, the programme is then spent and becomes worthless with no direction or purpose. In these rudderless situations we revert to type. And so the cycle continues. The solution to this issue is to find worth in the doing.

FINDING WORTH

When we outsource physical activity to machines it seems requisite we outsource a little common sense too. Consider this not unrealistic scenario: a man chooses to take the elevator over taking the stairs in order to reduce the activity cost of going up five storeys to his office. Later that day he chooses to drive to the gym instead of walking, again to reduce the physical cost. In the gym, he pays to use machines that replicate stair climbing and walking in order to increase his physical activity count for the day. Sounds crazy, right? It gets worse: earlier in the week he ordered firewood and paid extra to have it pre-chopped so that he could avoid the strenuous toil. Yet later in his workout he pays his personal trainer to teach him the correct technique for the "woodchopper" exercise using the cable machine.

Climbing the stairs to the office, walking from A to B, and chopping wood are activities that have worth. There is a reason for doing them, and there is a worthwhile output. When your physical activity is authentic and your efforts are productive it becomes a satisfying process. A process you can get lost in. And often it is free (you may even get paid to do it!). Instead, the prevailing fitness view is that we should look solely to gym-based exercise for our main source of physical activity. Unfortunately, this approach is largely devoid of any context and as such lacks intrinsic worth. So much so that we need distractions and extrinsic motivation to do it.

Take a moment to appraise your current exercise regimen. Do you enjoy it for what it is? Or do you endure it? Do you need to be distracted from it by conversation, music, podcasts, or television? Do you avoid it at every opportunity? Do you need someone to motivate you? Does it provide worth?

In order to add true worth to your activity it helps if it has a wider purpose. Our Paleolithic ancestors' physical activity provided food, shelter, security and warmth. Contrast that with what you do. If you were asked after your workout what you did, is your answer a series of numbers (I lifted X weight, Y times; I ran for X minutes at a heart rate of Y)? Or is the result of your toil real, such as a pile of chopped wood? Some more questions: is your physical activity useful? Does your fitness contribute anything? Could you help jump start a car? Leap a fence if a dog threatened to attack? If called upon, would you be useful in an emergency?

The solution is to integrate as much physical activity into your day in a way that has purpose to you and others. As we noted in Chapter One, tending a smallholding is physical activity that provides worth, in this case food. Appraise your day-to-day living and highlight where you have outsourced worthwhile physical activity, and reclaim as much of it as you can. Walk and take the stairs. Do your own housework rather than pay someone else to do it. Do your own D.I.Y. Chop your own wood; chop some for your neighbour while you are at it. Join the local beach clean. Be a useful, active human. You can measure the worth of your physical activity by its contribution.

AVOID THE TRAP

Gym-based exercises can be excellent for developing health and fitness, but if you are not careful they can become an end in themselves. Whilst the desire to improve at a particular exercise is laudable the process is not always so. Often the exercises become demonstrations of health and fitness rather than developing them. Continually striving to lift as much as possible in the bench press may seem a commendable goal, and continued improvement may be interpreted as an increase in health and fitness. This is an easy trap to fall into. This is an example of demonstrating strength, not necessarily developing it. The bench press is domain specific and makes you good at bench pressing. Fine if you are a powerlifter, but what if you are not? What value does it have outside of the gym?

It is important to note that the value does not always have to be quantifiable. Martial arts are an excellent means to develop mastery, where mastery is the worthwhile end goal; dance provides worth in its creative and expressive elements; team sports have worth in collaboration and bonding.

Arguably the best worth to get from your physical activity is enjoyment. And enjoyment should be regarded as a purpose in and of itself. Enjoyment is a key factor if physical activity is to become an integral part of your lifestyle. Most people dread going to the gym and regard it as a chore. It is therefore not surprising that most gym memberships go unused. If your physical activity does not have a wider purpose and you do not enjoy it, then it will not be sustainable for a lifetime. Your physical activity should be autotelic, where the goal is in the doing. It should be fun, just like it was when you played around as a kid.

And enjoyment does not necessarily mean it is easy, you can enjoy difficult too. You can hike harder trails, practice more challenging yoga poses, run some tougher hills. There is a crucial difference between pain and suffering. That difference is how you perceive it. By definition all hard physical work is painful, but if you enjoy it, it can bring a lot of pleasure, inspiration and reward. If you do not enjoy it, you will always feel like you are travailing.

Discipline

As we have previously noted, it is highly probable that even if you grasp every opportunity for incidental physical activity during your day, a shortfall will still remain when compared to the Ideal Physical Activity Profile (Figure 4, Chapter Four). This is the reality of modern living. And as we have seen, the remedy is resistance exercise. If you are not one of the fortunate who enjoy resistance exercise, you may find yourself in potential conflict: you need to do it, but you do not necessarily like it. Yes there is worth to it - it improves your health and fitness - but often these benefits are not immediate, and if you are not careful resistance exercise can become a grind, which is the very thing we want to avoid. In this book we have largely ameliorated the issue by using the brevity of the minimum effective load (Chapter Seven). Nonetheless, the exercises still need doing. This is where discipline comes in. Resistance exercise is a practice we must do if we want to maximise our longevity, and viewed through this lens it provides us with the opportunity to master discipline; a worthwhile trait to have.

Norman Mailer eruditely noted that, 'any workout which does not involve a certain minimum of danger or responsibility does not improve the body - it just wears it out.' It seems that somewhere along the way we have become distracted with gyms, machines and working out and as a result our physical activity has lost its context, meaning and purpose. So much so that working out has become an end in itself and even a chore to endure. I think the pioneering physical educator George Hébert provides us with best solution, 'be fit to be useful.' And the beauty is, being useful also makes us fit!

CHAPTER NINE: SPEND MORE TIME OUTDOORS

According to the United Nations, in 2008 we passed an unprecedented point in our hominid history; more of the human populous are now living in urban environments than outside of them. Think about that for a moment. It is a considerable social, environmental and lifestyle shift away from our natural environment. We are now living disconnected from our inherent biophilia, and this predicament is increasingly being linked to our ills.

The importance of the environment to our health is nothing new. Paracelsus, a 16th century philosopher and physician noted that, 'The art of healing comes from nature, not the physician. Therefore the physician must start from nature, with an open mind.' This concept of restoring vitality through nature has had long-standing intuitive appeal with many, but it has been notoriously difficult to quantify and assess. That is until relatively recently. Advances in psychology, neurosciences and our understanding of brain waves and stress hormones have enabled us to see how being in nature affects the function of our brains, our bodies, and our health. And these effects are now measurable. For example, walking for as little as 15 minutes in woodland has been shown to increase cognitive functioning, decrease the stress hormone cortisol, and reduce both heart rate and blood pressure. And in an ironic twist, it has been the development of technology, and in particular apps, that has enabled large-scale crowdsourced data to be collected and analysed by researchers. The findings are remarkably consistent: we are happy and feel invigorated when we are in nature.

GO GREEN

Independent research from across the globe is showing a common theme: the closer you live to green space the more positive your outlook will be, and the longer you can expect to live. This extended life comes with added benefits, such as: reduced stress and mental illness; lower incidences of asthma; lower blood pressure; lower levels of obesity, and an enhanced immune system to name a few. Of particular interest is the observation that you do not have to live in the countryside to profit from this effect; you can live in an urban area, and providing you have close proximity to urban green spaces (your street is tree lined or there are parks or woodland nearby) you can also reap these benefits.

Whilst the effects of green space on health are measurable, the mechanisms why are not so clear. An obvious answer is that those living near green spaces such as parks will use them and therefore exercise more, and it is the exercise not the green space per se that is providing the benefits. This is not necessarily the case; even those who live in close proximity to parks and do not use them, are also found to benefit.

One theory is that just viewing green space helps reduce stress. Neuroscience research is discovering that when people are shown pictures of urban environments the areas of their brains associated with fear and anxiety receive increased blood flow indicating greater activity, whereas when they are shown natural landscapes the areas of their brains associated with calmness receive more blood flow.

Urban dwellers experience chronic stress resulting from overcrowding, constant noise, air pollution, and continual distraction. In the Western world multitasking is seen as a laudable skill, whether in the office, at home or during recreation time. Our attention is continually distracted by, and divided among, several urgent demands to the extent that we are rarely fully absorbed in a single task and able to give it our full attention. This state pervades our entire waking day and is very demanding. Our brains, in particular the prefrontal cortex, can easily become fatigued. The prefrontal cortex is responsible for focusing attention and modulating complex behaviour, impulses and emotions. As you would expect it is on overdrive as a result of our highly stressful urban lives, and it negatively affects how we think, feel and behave. This attentional demand is not present in natural environments, and green spaces demand very little from us. It seems that nature is proving to be an antidote to the stress of urban living. It calms the mind, frees it from clutter and encourages a relaxed state. It puts us back in step with our natural surroundings and we think and feel better as a result. This is the basis of what psychologists call attention restoration theory.

Shinrin-yoku, or forest bathing, is now common practice in Japan as a form of preventative medicine, and the practice is spreading to the Western world. Forest bathing involves wandering in a green environment and engaging all of your senses in the experience and absorbing the natural atmosphere. When we are indoors we tend to have a hyper-focused, task-oriented attention. Whereas forest bathing encourages "soft fascination" such as when we watch wildlife or admire a view. Put another way, forest bathing provides room for our brains to wander off and recover. What urban environments deplete, nature helps restore.

Urban stress has a profound effect on our health and on the rate at which we age. Seminal research on patient recovery times and green space is compelling. Postoperative patients who have a window view looking out on nature have been shown to have faster recovery times and require fewer analgesics than those without the view. Similarly, residents of retirement homes report enhanced wellbeing if they have a room with a green view compared with those who do not.

BACK TO OUR ROOTS

Our ancestors' lives were completely immersed in the natural world, whereas nowadays we are increasingly spending more time indoors. Recent studies show that Westerners spend nearly 90 percent of the day in enclosed buildings shielded from nature. Lamentably, children's after school time is becoming increasingly scheduled with little time for outdoor free living. Even our physical activity is mostly inside. We are immersed in technology to such an extent that we now associate happiness and relaxation with the television. Our brains are processing different things when we are inside compared to when we are in green space.

Whether or not science has fully caught up with the underlying mechanisms is irrelevant. Being in nature makes us feel good and that is the main reason why we should do it. There is also intuitive appeal about the healing properties of the outdoors; it was in a natural environment where our senses evolved. It is the experience we were designed to experience.

Merely being in nature has a positive effect, but research is indicating that you can get increased benefit if you are active while you are there. This link between nature and health is so profound that physicians in New Zealand have been issuing "green prescriptions" to patients as a nationwide initiative for them to benefit from the synergy of being active in nature. One such benefit of us being active in a green environment is it increases our ventilation of fresh air which contains antimicrobial wood oils and phytoncides released by the flora. This in turn has been linked to many benefits including: lowering stress, reducing anxiety, and boosting the immune system, with the bonus that the effects can last for several weeks after the initial exposure.

BIG BLUE

Sea views always command a premium, whether you are booking a hotel room or a purchasing a beachfront house. And there is good reason. Notwithstanding the anxiety-inducing price tags, ocean views relieve stress and make us feel good. Researchers in this field call these views of open water "blue spaces" and they are finding evidence to support what we already feel; increasing exposure to blue space is associated with lower psychological stress and improved mental health. What better reason to justify the upgrade to an ocean view on your next holiday?

Being outside exposes us to different things compared with being indoors. We need some exposure to direct sunlight to stimulate the production of vitamin D. Our bodies require vitamin D to aid the absorption of phosphate and calcium from the foods that we eat. These minerals play important roles in maintaining healthy muscles, bones and teeth. A deficiency in vitamin D can lead to weak and deformed bones. Furthermore, a lack of vitamin D has been associated with increased risk of certain cancers, hypertension, heart disease and autoimmune dysfunction. Being outside also exposes us to dirt and animals, which researchers are finding may help develop and strengthen our immune systems. Again, this has intuitive appeal as we evolved and thrived in an environment surrounded by dirt and other animals.

SUNLIGHT EXPOSURE

Care must be exercised here as sunlight exposure is hormetic: too much and it is harmful to health, but so too is under exposure. However, there is a sweet spot that can be beneficial to health. But it is extremely important to remember that the strength of sunlight is different at different times of the day, and at different times of the year. It is also affected by where you are on Earth and your proximity to the equator. Furthermore, responses to sunlight are highly individualized and depend on skin type among other things. For these reasons it is prudent to seek the advice of your General Practitioner or Physician regarding the level of sun exposure that is beneficial for you.

CYCLICAL MOVEMENT

Our ancestors' activity profile was one of contrast. Hard physical work was followed by rest. Their work was varied and performed in accordance with the circadian light-dark cycle. Whereas, today's gym-based exercise tends to be repetitive (reps and sets) and performed at an intensity flatlined somewhere between hard and easy. Twenty-four-seven gyms and artificial lighting have further thrown ancestral activity patterns and circadian hormonal rhythms out of synchrony with the light-dark cycle. Scientists have known for some time that chronic disruption of circadian rhythms is harmful to health. It can negatively affect your immune system, mental health and even your lifespan.

In a wider context our ancestors' activity profile fluctuated with the seasons. Summer brought long daylight hours and prolonged activity with winter requiring less. Even in our recent past this was the case. Make hay while the sun shines was more than just an adage, it was a reality. Today we barely acknowledge the seasons when it comes to exercise. Personally, I prefer to exercise outdoors, and in doing so I cannot avoid the reality of the seasons. For me the summer brings more time for exercise and activity and with it a sense of space, time and creativity. The winter requires keeping active to stay warm, there is a sense of urgency and a need to get the job done. As such my exercise and activity patterns fluctuate in accordance with the seasons. Interestingly, modern athletic training shares similarities with this seasonal variation. In sports, the cycling of training emphasis and volume is known as periodization and it is the cornerstone of athletic programme design. Strength and conditioning coaches know that a constant training volume leads to boredom, overuse injuries, staleness and a lack of improvement.

Cycling our activity levels in accordance with the seasons has been part of hominid history for millennia and your health and fitness can benefit from this ancestral oscillation too. Whenever possible take your physical activity outdoors and reconnect with the seasonal periodization.

HYBRID THEORY

The association between nature and health and wellbeing is now well established. Yet sadly we are exposing ourselves less and less to green and blue spaces. Modern life is dominated with indoor living, often moving from one box to the next, with little time or thought for authentic interaction with nature. To some degree most people follow the modern box lifestyle (Figure 114).

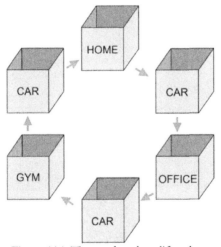

Figure 114: The modern box lifestyle

I am not suggesting that we ditch the modern world for a life off the grid, it is simply not realistic. However, once again the best solution is to have a hybrid approach so that we can maximize the gains from living in both the technological and natural worlds. We can use the trappings of technology to enhance our quality of life and also embrace the natural environment and its allied health benefits.

The positive response to nature is immediate and has a dose-response effect. None is bad for you, a little is better, and more is better still. Natural Resources Institute Finland are aware of this and recommend a minimum monthly dose of five cumulative hours to enhance wellbeing (this includes exposure to tree lined streets, weekend visits to parks, as well as prolonged trips in nature). This prescription is realistic for the vast majority of us, and is a worthwhile minimum to aim for.

Get outside as often as you can; morning and evening strolls are great ways to entrain your body to the light dark-cycle and get your circadian rhythms in tune with your environment. Whenever possible, perform your physical activity and resistance exercise in blue and green spaces. Bring nature into your workplace with house plants and pictures of natural landscapes. Be mindful and attend to the nature that surrounds you each and every day; even in cities there is an abundance of flora and fauna if you look for it. The nature solution is simple, it is easy, and it is free!

CHAPTER TEN:
NUTRITION

Nutrition can be a complex and emotive topic. It is also one of the most important. Get your nutrition right and a lot of things will fall into place, get it wrong and your efforts elsewhere will be largely wasted.

The reason for this complexity and emotivity is often down to the relationships we have with our food. On a biochemical level nutrition is pretty simple; the foods we consume provide us with the energy to live, and the building blocks for growth and repair. But when we move up to the human level, nutrition becomes multifactorial and complex. Consider for a moment your own relationship with food. What do you eat? Why do you eat? How do you eat? Where do you eat? When do you eat? With whom do you eat? There are many answers, and not all of them are good.

We can use food to create and maintain our identities. We can project wealth and sophistication based on where we choose to shop and dine. We can use food choices to express our views and morals. What we consume is heavily influenced by our education, understanding, beliefs, emotional state, inertia, finances, as well as the collective consciousness of peers, religion and media. And more often these days, what we eat is governed by how we want to look.

Things get more confusing when we add bad science and fad diets into the mix. These nostrums range from the somewhat plausible to the downright idiotic, but all fad diets tend to have one thing in common: they fail to work in the long-run. You may see some quick-fix benefits in the short-term, but few of them can be realistically sustained for a lifetime. Most are not nutritious and some are even harmful to your health.

Even amongst the experts there is a lack of agreement regarding the optimal diet. My goal for this chapter is not to add a further layer of complexity, or to prescribe a particular diet. That would be of little benefit. Instead my goal is actually the opposite; I want to simplify the process, promote mindful eating and give you the necessary tools to make informed choices.

In order to make sense out of this confusion, a good starting point is to return to our roots once more and seek guidance from our forebears' lifestyles to determine what we are genetically predisposed to consume and metabolize. In this chapter we shall explore whether it is possible, or even desirable for that matter, to recreate our ancestral diet.

WHAT DID OUR ANCESTORS EAT?

Information about the diet of Paleolithic humans comes mainly from the examination of coprolites (fossilized faeces) and skeletal remains. While this goes some way to aid our understanding of the dietary habits of our forebears it does not give us the full story, so to help complete the picture, information about the diets of contemporary hunters and gatherers is used.

It should be noted that even the diets of most modern hunters and gatherers have changed considerably from what our Paleolithic ancestors consumed, in particular the type and availability of food. Unfortunately, most modern tribespeople have been marginalized to relatively unforgiving territories (typically: the arctic, deserts, and tropical forests) where lands are less fertile and uncultivated plants are less bountiful. Furthermore, the variety and availability of wild game is far less now than it was in Paleolithic times. Back then the human population was considerably smaller and the population of game was far greater. Even in relatively recent history, explorers charting the New World would often comment on the abundance and diversity of game.

Contemporary tribespeople are also more technologically developed than our early Paleolithic ancestors. Even a simplistic tool like the bow and arrow was invented relatively recently (circa late upper Paleolithic to Mesolithic). These tools will clearly affect the type of game that can be hunted. And there are few remaining tribes that have not had a degree of influence from the outside world and adopted at least some of our modern tools. Nonetheless, the lifestyles of modern hunters and gatherers are as close to those of the Paleolithic tribespeople as we are going to get and observations of their lifestyle can go some way to inform us of our dietary heritage. By its very nature, this approach produces generalisations and with it has come substantial disagreement among the experts in the field. As such the information should be viewed and interpreted accordingly.

OUR PALEOLITHIC ANCESTORS' DIETS

It is worth noting here that I have referred to Paleolithic diets (plural) rather than the popular term "Paleo diet" (singular). The reason is many diets existed back then. Humans have, and still do, thrive in vastly different ecosystems ranging from arid deserts to high altitude mountainous regions and everything in between. The Paleolithic period was the longest in our history spanning approximately 2.5 million years. During this time humans existed in different climates and environments and during great feast and famine periods.

We only have to look at the diets of two contemporary tribes for examples of diversity. For Inuit tribes living in the arctic, where flora is scarce, around 95% of their calories come from meat (mainly fish and sea mammals), whereas for the !Kung people living in the Kalahari Desert only about 10% of their calories come from meat with the majority coming from seeds, nuts and plants. These are clearly widely different dietary practises yet both groups thrive. If nothing else, this tells us the human body did not evolve to be sustained by a single diet, instead it is extremely flexible and we can thrive on a variety of foods. We have evolved to be generalist omnivores. The corollary therefore is an optimal diet does not exist.

CAN THE PALEOLITHIC DIETS BE REPLICATED?

The answer is no. Simply put there are now too many of us, and too few wild game, for everyone to eat like our Paleolithic ancestors. Furthermore, animals and plants that exist now are different than they were back then. Many of the animals our pre-agricultural ancestors consumed, such as giant sloths, mammoths and woolly rhinoceros are now extinct. And a lot of the ones that are still around such as bison and deer are rarely found in our butchers or supermarkets.

As a result of domestication and genetic selection our Neolithic and more recent ancestors were able to breed animals with desirable characteristics such as plumpness and docility. Efficient animals that are capable of rapid weight gain have been prized, so too has tender meat rather than the tough wild variety. Over time the gulf between wild and domesticated animals became wide and has widened considerably over the last century or so following the introduction of scientific breeding and feeding practices. Grain, antibodies and hormones are typically used to facilitate this process.

Plants have had a similar fate. Only a select few were chosen to be cultivated to maximize yield, with the majority being abandoned. These chosen floras have been altered to reduce seed content and naturally occurring toxins (for example, Paleolithic beans contained cyanide), whilst the size of kernels, fruits and the amount of flesh have been enhanced. Cultivated nuts and beans now have thinner shells making them more accessible. We could probably still recognize some of the fruits from Paleolithic times, although back then they tended to be smaller and tarter than their modern descendants. However, the Paleolithic vegetables are a different story, chances are we would not recognize them at all. They were small, contained little flesh and were woody, tough and fibrous. Brussels sprouts, broccoli, collard greens, cauliflower and kale did not even exist back then, they are cultivators of a single species of wild cabbage (brassica oleracea), such is our ability to genetically select and cultivate.

A RETURN TO THE SEASONS

Our deep ancestors clearly had no other option than to eat what was available in their immediate geographic location. Their diet was further influenced by seasonal variation. However, we have since mastered our environment to such an extent that we can get whatever food we desire from anywhere in the world whenever we want it. No longer do we have to wait for the appropriate season to eat a particular food; we are living in the age of the year-round strawberry! You could be forgiven for thinking that this increased bandwidth is a good thing and that it would lead to a more diverse and nutritious diet. Interestingly, this does not seem to be the case. Instead, we tend to limit our food choices to just our favourites, which we then consume week in, week out. When it comes to food we are creatures of habit.

A problem with this homogenous eating preference is it bypasses seasonal rhythm, and in doing so ignores the intimate and important relationship between seasonal food and seasonal activity. Summer brings long daylight hours and provides the opportunity and inclination for prolonged physical activity. Mother nature matches this with a carbohydrate-rich summer harvest. And as we all know, autumn and winter bring shorter, colder days during which we are less inclined to get outside and be active. This is naturally in step with the wintertime harvest with its warming, protein and fat-rich produce. This harmony should not be surprising; human evolution and pre-human evolution were forged in a seasonal crucible. Only recently have we divorced ourselves from the Earth's changing position in relation to the sun.

Over the long-term, seasonal eating provides a wide variety of micro nutrients at different times of the year, and in doing so prevents malnutrition and avoids toxicity. The heavy, high-fat, high-protein winter harvest provides certain key nutrients, but it also has the potential to allow fat soluble toxins to accumulate. The proceeding low-fat, low-calorie spring harvest provides additional nutrients, helps detoxify the winter accumulation and prepares the body for the summer.

Each seasonal harvest naturally has a different emphasis: spring foods promote low-fat, low-calorie eating; summer is a high-carbohydrate harvest; and the autumn/winter harvest is a bounty of high-fat and high-protein foods. Taken individually it is easy to see the similarities between each seasonal harvest and contemporary vogue diets. Spring is similar to the classic weight loss diet, summer resembles the typical athletic diet, and the popular "Paleo" diet echoes the autumn/winter harvest.

The important and critical difference between seasonal eating and fad diets is the latter recommend continual adherence with no concern for seasonal rhythm. If we view these fad diets through a seasonal lens, it becomes clear why some people may have success with them in the short-term but not the long-term. Any short-lived success of a fad diet will depend upon the time of the year it was adopted. If a weight-loss diet is adopted in the spring, the initial results are likely to be positive, but they will soon wane as the season changes. Whereas if it is adopted in the winter, any early success would likely be blunted. Furthermore, when a fad diet is adopted it is likely there will be some initial benefits resulting from the introduction of the nutrients that were previously absent. However, continual adherence to the new diet will likely expose deficiencies in other nutrients which are now not present. This may also go someway to explain why scientific endeavours to determine the efficacy of certain diets is equivocal; more often than not the research methodologies do not take time of year and seasonal variation into account and few studies are of sufficient length to expose the limitations of continual adherence.

SEASONAL FOODS
Eating seasonally should enable you to buy local (though it is okay to include foods from the same season grown in other parts of the world). This is not only good for the local economy, but it also means the produce is fresher because transit and storage times are less. It is even better if you can purchase your food at source from farmers' markets as this gives you the opportunity to ask the farmers directly about their husbandry and make your food choices accordingly. Seasonal foods can be grouped according to the main growing and harvest seasons. For the vast majority of our hominid history there was no other option than to eat in accordance with the seasons. This has been recognized in Ayurvedic medicine for centuries. The growing/harvest seasons are: Spring (March – June); Summer (July – October); Autumn/Winter (November – February). Personally, I feel that seasonal food tastes better and that foods from the same season compliment each other. Below are some common foods categorized by season (note: this corresponds to the UK harvests and is not an exhaustive list).

SPRING (March - June)
Following the high-fat, high-protein and low-metabolic winter, the spring naturally provides a low-fat harvest, which coaxes the body to favour using stored fat as an energy source. Body fat is where toxins accumulate, so as the body fat is metabolized during the spring the toxins are released and eliminated from the body. Bitter greens such as rocket make up the spring harvest which help the liver cleanse the body of impurities. Spring can be viewed as nature's detox season.

Fish
Cockles, cod, coley, crab, dab, Dover sole, gurnard, haddock, hake, halibut, herring, John Dory, langoustine, lemon sole, lobster, mussels, oysters, plaice, pollack, prawns, red mullet, salmon, sardines, scallops, sea bream, sea trout, shrimp, squid, whelks, whitebait, winkle.

Fruits
Apricots, bananas, bilberries, blood oranges, blueberries, cherries, gooseberries, grapefruit, greengages, kiwi fruit, lemons, limes, oranges, passion fruit, peaches, pineapple, rhubarb, strawberries.

Herbs
Basil, chamomile, chervil, chives, coriander, dill, elderflower, mint, nasturtium, oregano, parsley, rosemary, sage, sorrel, summer savory, tarragon, thyme.

Meat
Beef, chicken, duck, lamb, wood pigeon.
Vegetables
Artichoke, asparagus, aubergine, beetroot, broad beans, broccoli, carrots, cauliflower, chillies, courgettes, fennel, French beans, garlic, kale, kohlrabi, leeks, lettuce, mangetout, new potatoes, onions, pak choi, peas, purple sprouting broccoli, radishes, rocket, runner beans, salad leaves, salsify, samphire, savoy cabbage, spinach, spring onions, swede, tomatoes, turnips, watercress, wild nettles.

SUMMER (July - October)

The summer harvest is dominated by carbohydrate-rich fruits and vegetables. These naturally provide the energy to match our higher levels of physical activity in the summer. We also need more fluids at this time of year, and consuming water-rich foods such as courgettes and cucumbers helps us maintain our hydration levels.

Fish
Clams, cod, coley, crab, dab, Dover sole, grey mullet, gurnard, haddock, hake, halibut, herring, langoustine, lemon sole, lobster, mackerel, monkfish, mussels, oysters, pilchard, plaice, pollack, prawns, red mullet, sardines, scallops, sea bass, sea bream, sea trout, shrimp, skate, sole, squid, turbot, whelks, whitebait, wild salmon, winkles.

Fruits
Apples, apricots, bilberries, blackberries, blueberries, cherries, damsons, elderberries, figs, gooseberries, grapes, greengages, kiwi fruit, loganberries, medlar, melons, nectarines, peaches, pears, plums, quince, raspberries, redcurrants, strawberries.

Grains
Barley.

Herbs
Basil, chervil, chives, coriander, dill, elderflowers, oregano, mint, nasturtium, parsley, rosemary, sage, sorrel, tarragon, thyme.

Meat
Beef, duck, goose, grouse, guinea fowl, hare, lamb, mallard, partridge, pheasant, rabbit, turkey, venison, wood pigeon.

Nuts
Almonds, chestnuts, hazelnuts, walnuts.

Vegetables
Artichoke, aubergine, beetroot, broad beans, broccoli, butternut squash, carrots, cauliflower, celeriac, celery, chillies, courgettes, cucumbers, fennel, French beans, garlic, horseradish, Jerusalem artichoke, kale, kohlrabi, leeks, lettuce, mangetout, marrow, new potatoes, onions, pak choi, parsnips, peas, peppers (sweet), potatoes, pumpkin, radishes, rocket, runner beans, salad

leaves, salsify, samphire, shallots, spinach, spring onions, swede, sweetcorn, tomatoes, turnips, watercress, wild nettles.

AUTUMN/WINTER (November - February)

As we move into autumn and winter our appetite for raw salads and vegetables wanes and instead we crave fortifying soups and stews. During this season the availability of carbohydrate-rich fruits is less, instead heavy, warming root vegetables are harvested and we rely more on protein and fat-rich foods such as grains, nuts and meats. The winter diet is naturally high in protein and fat which help keep us warm and nourished through the colder months.

Fish
Clams, cod, coley, crab, dab, Dover sole, gurnard, haddock, hake, halibut, langoustine, lemon sole, lobster, mackerel, monkfish, mussels, oysters, plaice, pollack, red mullet, scallops, sea bass, sea bream, skate, squid, turbot, winkles.

Fruits
Apples, bananas, blood oranges, clementines, cranberries, kiwi fruit, lemons, oranges, passion fruit, pears, pineapples, pomegranate, quince, rhubarb, satsumas, tangerines.

Grains
Barley, oats, wheat.

Herbs
Basil, parsley, rosemary, sage, savory.

Meat
Beef, chicken, duck, goose, grouse, guinea fowl, hare, lamb, mallard, partridge, pheasant, pork, rabbit, turkey, venison, wood pigeon.

Nuts
Almonds, hazelnuts, chestnuts, walnuts

Vegetables
Artichoke, beetroot, broccoli, brussels sprouts, butternut squash, cabbage, cauliflower, celeriac, celery, chicory, horseradish, Jerusalem artichoke, kale, kohlrabi, leeks, parsnips, potatoes (maincrop), pumpkin, purple sprouting broccoli, salsify, shallots, swede, truffles (black), truffles (white), turnips, watercress, wild mushrooms.

TIMING IS EVERYTHING

When you eat can be just as important as what you eat. From an athletic standpoint we are all familiar with the concept of allowing the muscular system, or the cardiovascular system, a period of recovery following a bout of exercise stress. Repetitive exercise bouts with insufficient rest can lead to overtraining and burnout. The digestive system is no different; it too requires regular periods of rest in order to function optimally.

A corollary of our diurnal lifestyle is a fasting period of about eight hours when we sleep. However, this rest period is only of benefit to the digestive system if we avoid eating late in the evening. A late main meal may still be getting processed throughout the night, forcing the digestive system to work at a time when it should be recovering.

In order to maximize this digestive rest period it helps to extend the night-time fast. This can be achieved by having the last meal of the day (we shall call it dinner) as early as possible, say around 6.00 pm and having breakfast (breaking the fast) as late as possible, let's say 10.00 am. This equates to a fast of around sixteen hours. These bookend meals should be small and light, with the most substantial meal of the day being lunch.

The early morning is the body's time for the elimination of waste, not digestion. A late, light breakfast, preferably after some light morning exercise, will gently ease the digestive system into the day. A large lunch should provide the bulk of the energy and nutrients needed for the rest of the day, and it is consumed at the time when the digestive system functions best. Lunch should be followed by an easy-paced ten-minute stroll. An early, light dinner helps the digestive system wind down before bedtime. This routine reduces the night-time digestive stress and enables the body to focus on what it should be doing: recovery, repair and detoxification.

Timing meals to ensure a significant fasted period is known as time restricted eating. When you eat has a powerful influence on your digestive circadian rhythm, which in turn influences the functioning of your body's other systems. The moment you break the night-time fast signals when your digestive system is open for business and the clock starts ticking. You have a 12 hour window during which your digestive system is working at its best, so you should aim to eat your last meal within this timeframe to take full advantage (current research is showing that an eight to ten hour window is optimal). It is important that you are consistent with the timing of your meals, especially breakfast, in order to optimally entrain your digestive circadian rhythm.

Our modern lifestyles are not very accommodating of this style of eating. Nowadays most of us work in offices, service industries or factories, and lunchtimes tend to be brief and are often used to run errands. Here food is a second thought, consumed on the run or while multitasking. This hectic lifestyle necessitates an early and more substantial breakfast (it is worth noting that the 'breakfast-like-a-king' philosophy is only a modern construct) with the main meal getting knocked back to later in the evening. Both of these times are when food is poorly digested. In order to maintain waning energy levels during the day there is a need for continual grazing, which unfortunately keeps the digestive system working. This may go some way to explain the prevalence of indigestion and other gastric issues that we see today.

Get real!

I am guessing that there are two issues that have jumped out at you with regard to time restricted eating. Firstly, you are probably thinking that you would be left hungry with a light, late breakfast and a light, early dinner. And secondly you are probably concerned that it would be very difficult to fit a large meal in at lunchtime.

It is important to note that the total amount of food you consume is not reduced so you should not go hungry; it's only the timing and emphasis that are altered. If you are running out of energy it is likely you are not eating enough for your lunch. Finding time for this large lunch during the working week is effortful at first. To make time restricted eating work you will have to make your digestive system your number one priority. Weekends are a good place to start as you probably have more control over them. Then aim for an additional day during the working week, then two and so on. If you decide to adopt this eating pattern, you are also going to have to come up with coping strategies. You will probably need to prepare your food in advance. At work, you may need to get off site so you are not disturbed by colleagues or emails. And you may have to get uber organized with your personal admin so that you can avoid using your lunchtime for other tasks.

This may seem onerous, but like with most things if you stick with it over time it will become habitual. That said, do not get hung up if you cannot adhere to it all of the time. Just observing the broad principles helps. Even if you can only be consistent with the timing of your breakfast, or you just eat your evening meal a little earlier, each gesture means your digestive system will be getting a little help, and it will thank you for it!

PROCESSING

All food requires some form of processing before we eat it. At one end of the continuum there is minimal processing, such as picking and peeling a banana, where the nutritional content is essentially left unchanged. And at the other end there are foodstuffs that have undergone considerable processing, such as fast food and confectionery, where the nutritional content has been lessened considerably. Most authorities on nutrition agree that minimal processing is best and highly processed foods should be avoided.

Our early ancestors ate their food raw or following only minimal processing. Their processing methods were limited to scraping, pounding, baking and roasting. These are healthy processing methods and the foods tend to retain the majority of their fibre and nutrients. In contrast, modern methods of food processing strip our foods of a lot of their nutrients and add ingredients (fat, sugar, preservatives and other chemicals) which can be harmful to health. Below are some tips to clean up and improve your diet.

TIPS FOR INTEGRATING A HEALTHY DIET INTO YOUR LIFESTYLE
Purge the processed food
If you accept that processed food is not good for you, then you have no further need for it. Get rid of it. Literally. Avoid the temptation to finish off what is in the cupboards as this action continues to condone the consumption of

processed food and delays the transition to a healthier diet. Consider donating
your discarded food to your local food bank to help those less fortunate.

Shop locally and seasonally
Now it is time to get your new supplies in and fill your fridge and cupboards
with unprocessed food. Only buy from stores that have a quick turnover of
fresh produce, the longer it is on the shelves the more it is degrading. Get into
the habit of shopping frequently and only purchasing what you know you will
consume immediately. If buying fresh is not always possible, frozen and canned
vegetables (no sugar or salt added) are great staples to get in. Studies have
shown that produce can lose nearly half its essential nutrients by the time it
reaches our tables. The journey from farm to table can take as long as two weeks
exposing the produce to heat and light along the way, factors which reduce
freshness and nutritional value. Frozen fruit and vegetables are often frozen
within a few hours of being harvested, essentially preserving the freshness and
nutrient content of the produce. Fish is similar, opt for canned or frozen wild
varieties if you cannot buy locally sourced catches.

Expand your palate
If we view food as letters of the alphabet, it follows that the more varied your
diet, the more letters of the alphabet you have at your disposal and the more
words you can construct. Thus a limited diet would restrict your vocabulary.
Similarly, if the various processes of your body require building blocks derived
from your food, it follows that the greater the variety of building blocks in your
diet, the better able your body is to build and maintain itself. In light of this,
challenge yourself to try a new in-season fruit or vegetable each week.

One ingredient
A simple way to clean up your diet is to go with the "one ingredient" approach.
When purchasing your food aim to select those that only have one ingredient.
This practice will help you distinguish between food and food products. Of
course later you can make meals from combining these single ingredients. This
way you have control of what goes into the dish. You have little control with
multi-ingredient processed foods.

80:20 quality principle
A lot of things in life fall into the 80:20 principle or Pareto distribution. If you
are not familiar with it, the principle states that 80 percent of your outcomes
come from 20 percent of your inputs. And generally your diet is no different.
You will no doubt consume 20 percent of the foods you eat per season 80
percent of the time. In other words, you will have staple seasonal foods. This
being the case it makes sense to ensure these are the best quality they can be.
Deduce what they are by performing a simple diet audit and then aim to make
them the best quality you possibly can.

Choose well
✓ Choose food over food products
✓ Choose local, seasonal produce
✓ Choose wild over farmed
✓ Choose organic over conventional farming methods
✓ Choose free range over caged
✓ Choose grass fed over grain fed
✓ Choose whole over pre-cut produce and do not peel or chop anything until it is ready to use

---

GO ORGANIC
There is much debate over the nutritional content of organic produce compared to those subject to intensive farming methods. However, even if organic produce is not nutritionally superior, it is not exposed to the chemicals, antibiotics and exogenous hormones used in standard farming and thus do not contain the residues of these toxins. For this reason alone, it makes sense to choose organic.

Often organic food will cost more, and this is where the 80:20 principle really helps. It would be great if all of your nutrition was organic, however the associated increase in cost might be significant. Instead only 20 percent of the range of your food per season needs to be organic as you will consume it 80 percent of the time. This enables you to buy in bulk (and freeze) and thus cut down on costs. Of course the remaining 80 percent should still be the best quality possible and predominantly adhere to the bullet points above.

In reality I have not experienced a significant increase in the cost of eating organic especially when I view my grocery bill as a whole. Whilst organic items may cost a little more than their non-organic counterparts, you will no doubt find that when you eat clean you buy fewer items. By this I mean there will be less alcohol and confectionery in your shopping basket and you will be less inclined to have a pastry with your mid-morning coffee at work. As such your overall weekly spend will probably not be that much different.

Develop your cooking skills
If you do not already do so, start cooking your own meals. Again you can take advantage of the 80:20 principle here. In the beginning you only need to learn how to prepare 20 percent of the range of your meals per season and you will have 80 percent of what you eat covered. Preparing your own meals increases your relationship and knowledge of the foods you are eating. You are in control and can make tweaks to the ingredients to maximize the nutritious content of what you are consuming. The easiest way to do this is to search the Internet for healthy recipes of your favourite meals. Over time you can increase your repertoire of meals that you can prepare. Furthermore, if you experiment with a different food each week you will need to know how to prepare and cook it.

Prepare in bulk

Spontaneous eating is synonymous with poor nutrition. This is especially so if we leave it until we are hungry to make our decision. Prepare your meals in bulk and freeze them and you will always have a nutritious meal to hand. It also saves a lot of time; making one big chilli takes the same time as making a small one, yet provides several meals. You can buy ingredients in bulk which means food is cheaper. And with a freezer full of a variety of good quality meals you are less likely to be caught out when your schedule is busy (this will also help with the logistics of ensuring you have a large lunch).

Do not count the calories, make the calories count

In a similar vein to the fiscal advice "take care of the pennies and the pounds will look after themselves," so too with calories. Get the quality, timing and motivation of your diet sorted and the calories will take care of themselves. These days it seems that calories are the driving force at the expense of quality. Instead concern yourself with choosing real, good quality food. Foods are synergistic and work together; they are so much more than just their calorie content. Contemporary research in nutrigenomics is revealing how the foods we eat interact with our genes. Poor nutrition can negatively affect gene function leading to health issues, whereas quality nutrition boosts health and robustness.

Feed your brain

Take an active interest in your nutritional understanding. Read around the subject, take on board what makes sense, reject what does not and continuously update and enhance your diet.

Be mindful

Nutrition is often habitual. Make the shift from mindless eating to being mindful about what you consume and why.

Stay in control

You are in control of you. The choices are yours. Be creative and purposeful with your eating habits. And always, always enjoy your food.

BODY WEIGHT MAINTENANCE

Our ancestors evolved in an environment where food was not as caloric or as easily available as it is today. As such, being hardwired to crave high-energy food like fats and sugars was a very good adaptation to promote survival. So too were the propensities to avoid unnecessary activity and to readily store excess energy as body fat. Due to the physical work needed to acquire food, and the lower caloric content of our ancestors' diets, becoming obese or developing type II diabetes was not an issue for them. As such our evolution did not involve any compensatory adaptations to deal with the environment of pizzas, confectionery, sugary drinks and minimal physical activity that we find ourselves in today. Unfortunately, we have the same innate drivers regarding food and activity that our ancestors did.

Evidence suggests that our Paleolithic ancestors consumed about 3000 kcal a day. The UK National Health Service recommends that a healthy male requires 2500 kcal to maintain his weight. If our healthy male was to engage in physical activity, he would require further energy consumption which would bring the figure closer to that of his Paleolithic comparison. The agreement between these figures should not be surprising as we are dealing with members of the same species, the only difference is they are separated by millennia.

However, current estimates of the daily energy content of the Western diet is over 3400 kcal for the UK and over 3700 kcal for the USA. It should come as no surprise therefore that due to the excess consumption of calories, two thirds of adults in these countries are overweight or obese. This is an important lesson for us all: we tend to overeat.

The body weight of our pre-agricultural ancestors was fairly stable with only slight seasonal variations of about 3 to 5 percent. This is similar for modern hunter and gatherer tribes. Over the course of a year the losses and gains balance out and do not result in the year-on-year weight gain that we observe in Western societies.

If you are currently overweight, adopting the tenets of this book (eating unprocessed, seasonal food at the correct time of day allied to a movement-rich lifestyle) should be all you need to do to lose weight and establish your ideal, stable body weight. However, if you are practising the above and are still finding it difficult to lose weight, it may be that you are eating too much. It is important to note that there is a biological lag between consuming food and your brain registering how full you are. If you rush your meals you may have overeaten by the time you feel full. Research has shown that there can be up to 1000 kcal difference between feeling satisfied and feeling full. To give your brain the time it needs to measure your satiety, eat mindfully, slow down your eating, thoroughly chew your food and savour your meals. We can learn a lot from the Japanese practice hara hachi bu, which means "eat until you are 80 percent full." The Okinawan people of Japan embrace this approach to eating and are famous for having one of the highest rates of centenarians in the world, they suffer a fraction of the diseases associated with modern lifestyles and have more healthy years of life.

FOOD FOR THOUGHT
The Western diet is considerably different from that of our forebears. For optimal health and vitality it makes sense for us to move our diet back into the range that we are genetically adapted for. As we have seen, we cannot match like for like, but we can aim for a twenty first century diet that has a similar nutritional quantity and range as that of our Paleolithic ancestors. To summarize, the triad principles of sound nutrition are:

✓ Eat local, seasonal produce
✓ Avoid processed foods
✓ Eat at the correct time

As we have noted, there is no such thing as a single optimal diet for a human. We can thrive on a wide range of foods. What's more, each of us responds differently to different foods. The best diet for you, is the healthiest one that you can live with. You will know if your diet is working if:

✓ You do not get ill often
✓ You are not overweight
✓ Your skin is clear
✓ You do not have excessive wind
✓ You have regular bowel movement
✓ Your teeth and gums are healthy
✓ You feel energized
✓ You enjoy it!

CHAPTER ELEVEN: TRIBE

Humans cannot exist in a vacuum, we need each other to survive and thrive. Down through the ages we have worked collaboratively as tribes and it has helped us achieve more than we ever could have on our own; hunting game required the cooperation of other humans to achieve as a group what an individual could not. And game provided sustenance for the whole group.

Interaction and cooperation is good for us; it expands our understanding, develops our creativity, and provides us with that special sense of belonging that acts as a buffer from daily stress. But as we shall soon see, our tribe can also be our nemesis; being with the wrong group can reduce our life experiences, our health and ultimately our longevity.

IT IS GOOD TO BE WANTED
Our social interdependencies and our ability to cooperate mean humans have become a superorganism. We are a collective and we need each other. Our Paleolithic forebears would have spent their entire lives in the company of others. There would have been few occasions when they were truly alone. As a corollary, their choices and actions would have had the common good of the group at heart over self-interest.

It is not uncommon in Western society to live and work among strangers. Within the family unit, parents often commute (sometimes considerable distances) to work away from their family tribe. And for large portions of the day, children are brought up and educated by strangers. Moreover, in Western society the emphasis has moved away from the success of the tribe towards the performance and success of the individual. This approach is typical of education, careers and sports. Today we are assessed on our individual merits. We are measured with exam grades, performance targets, and our ability to best a fellow human. And we continually dance with the spectre of being dispensable if we fail to perform. This has become so important in our lives that often we have little time for family and friends and sadly they have become collateral damage. This is at odds with our ancestral living where each member of the tribe was valued and contributed to the whole.

STAYING ALIVE

For our distant ancestors, being part of a social network was a key aspect of staying alive. Being ostracized was an extremely treacherous situation to be in and without the synergistic and protective benefits of the tribe the predicament was often fatal. If our ancestors found themselves in isolation, their vigilance was on chronic overdrive. This is a highly stressful and enervating situation to be in. Even today, when thankfully the consequences of being ostracized are not immediately life threatening, this social artefact from our ancient past lives on in us, and it helps explain why we all seek social acceptance.

A key component of a happy and healthy life is feeling connected to other humans. This intrinsic need is independent of extrinsic factors such as how we look, what car we drive, or our job status or our salary. Our Paleolithic ancestors no doubt had a similar gamut of emotions as we do today, they will have experienced: hopes, fears, desires, sadness, joy, and stress. However, they would not have had to deal with any of these alone. Today, social isolation is endemic and loneliness is a known contributor to poor mental health. It comes as no surprise that increased prevalence of mental health issues goes hand in hand with increased urbanisation.

COLD COMFORT

One of the great success stories of our modernisation is we have made our environment safe. The vast majority of us can go about our daily business content in the knowledge that we are being looked after by our emergency services and armed forces. This is such a privileged position to be in. But it does come at a price. We are no longer faced with the visceral challenges of survival. Most of us live our entire lives cosseted; we always have a roof over our heads and food in our bellies. We never face danger and our mettle has never been, nor will it ever be, tested. We have never truly relied on anyone else for our survival and never had to come to the aid of a fellow in danger. We no longer have skin in the game.

Visceral reliance on each other is no more acute than during the aftermath of a large-scale disaster. Catastrophes expose the ephemeral worth of extrinsic success and self-interest; what matters is what each member can do for the group. Interestingly survivors of disasters and wars often reminisce favourably about the tribe mentality and the special bonds created when everyone is pulling together for the benefit of the group. Sadly, this soon dissipates when the threat is over.

IT IS A SMALL WORLD

It is a small world as the saying goes. And indeed it is. The parlour game Six Degrees of Separation posits that every person on the planet can be connected to every other person via six or fewer links in a chain. The links of the chain being, a friend, a friend's friend, a friend's friend's friend, and so on. Early academic inquiry found that the Six Degrees of Separation concept was indeed true. If a participant was asked to post a letter to a stranger elsewhere in the world (whose address was unkown), it could be successfully delivered to the recipient by forwarding the letter through a network of friends and friends' friends within six links of the chain. This simple experiment highlights the larger interconnected social web that we are all part of. And this social web has far reaching effects on how we live. Your social network influences, among other things: the way you think and behave, your beliefs and values, the music you listen to, and even your next online purchase. And it also has a dramatic influence on your health.

Choose your friends wisely

In regard to guaranteeing a successful start in life, the philosopher Bertrand Russell is credited with the pithy phrase, 'choose your parents wisely'. This aptly summarizes the influence genetics and upbringing have on our lives. However, it would appear that our health and longevity are not only affected by our familial genetics and lifestyle, but also dependent on the genetics and life choices of our friends, and our friends' friends, and our friends' friends' friends. Our social networks are crucial to our health.

In our deep past when we were out hunting it was imperative that key information was spread throughout the tribe rapidly and silently; if not starvation and death could result. If a tribe member noticed a predator ahead, it would have taken too long to explain this perilous situation to each member of the tribe in turn. Furthermore, during the retelling, the message could easily have become corrupt and spread confusion among the group. Moreover, the verbal communication may have alerted the predator to the tribe's presence. In situations like this, the safest and most efficient way to communicate is via the emotions. To do this effectively, each member of the group needs to be deft at reading and mimicking each other. This is something we have evolved to be adroit at and it is still with us today. We intensely observe emotions and behaviours in others and can interpret them in an instant; you know immediately when you enter a room whether the vibe is mellow or hostile.

Being able to read each other is also a key part of fitting in and being diplomatic in our relationships. If we can interpret others' behaviours and copy them we are more likely to be accepted. Interestingly mimicking can be a conscious or unconscious act, which suggests we may not be in complete control of our own behaviour, even though we may think we are.

Academics have known for some time that behaviours are contagious within groups and often spread in a similar fashion to communicable diseases. Recent studies are finding that obesity spreads through a population in this way too. At first this may seem implausible as obesity is not infectious, but the data show that if your best friend becomes obese the chances of you also becoming obese is nearly threefold that if your friend remained at his, or her, normal weight. Other patterns are observable too, for example normal weight individuals are more likely to have normal weight friends, whose friends and whose friends' friends are also normal weight. Whereas obese individuals tend to have a social network dominated by obese people. A plausible explanation for this observation might be that physically fit people (who are likely to be normal weight) go to the same gym and wind up as friends, similarly it might be that people who like a particular fast food restaurant hang out there and become friends and gain weight. It may also be that we simply like to hang around with people who are similar to us, a social phenomenon called homophily.

A further explanation for the widespread transmission of obesity from person to person within a social group is a change in normative values. If the people with whom you surround yourself with all gain weight, it will affect what you perceive as a normal acceptable body size. Indeed to fit in with the group you may, consciously or unconsciously, adopt the eating habits and expectations of the group. A good example of this passive normative acceptance is how it is generally assumed that as we age we will put weight on. Gaining body weight as we age is not a biological blueprint, rather it is a sociological norm. But because it happens to the vast majority of the population we take it for granted that it is just a normal part of getting old.

KNOW YOUR ONIONS

If you view your social circle as layers of an onion, the more layers you are surrounded by that hold the same values, the more likely you are to adopt those values, and the more difficult it is to rid yourself of them. The health of the people we have in our social network has a considerable influence over our own health. Furthermore, you do not have to know the people in the network to be influenced by them. This phenomenon, known as hyperdyadic spread, even extends to your friends' friends' friends. For example, your friend's colleagues, whom you may never meet, may influence your friend who in turn influences you. This social network branches out like the limbs of a tree, and you only have to get to the third degree of separation to have an awful lot of people all having an influence on your health. Furthermore, even strangers who exist outside of your wider social network can influence your behaviour. Research suggests that if you are at a buffet and are seated next to a stranger who is a big eater, there is an increased likelihood you will unwittingly select a larger portion for yourself.

It is highly likely that the power of the social network is a contributing factor as to why most attempts at lifestyle change fail in the long-term. If you are a sole dieter in a social group whose members are overweight, to succeed you must actively avoid the behaviours of the group and risk being ostracized. This is exactly the sort of thing we are hardwired not to do; our factory setting is to copy the group. To maintain this opposing behaviour indefinitely would be extremely tiring and stressful, and there may simply be too much social pressure to revert to the behaviours of the group and fit in. And this is what we observe time and time again. Yo-yo dieting, ineffective health promotion initiatives, and repeated failed attempts to get fit, serve as examples here.

Of course there is a flipside and you can benefit from social norms too. The good news is social contagion can work positively. If your friends and their friends and their friends adopt healthy behaviours, such as quitting smoking or increasing physical activity, then the likelihood is you will adopt these behaviours too. If your goal is to eat healthily and you join a group where the norm is healthy living the social pressures are now in your favour to succeed. Happiness and positivity have also been found to spread in a similar way. Interestingly, those communities where people live the longest and are most healthy foster values where healthy behaviours are the norm.

The power of your social network to influence your behaviour should not be underplayed. It is unsettling, but you do not have full control over what you do. The central concept of this book is about changing how we live in order to become healthier. However, if this is done deep within a social network that does not adopt the new behaviours it can make the change extremely difficult, if not impossible.

In order to give yourself the best chance of succeeding at making healthy lifestyle choices, you can stack the odds in your favour by using this understanding of social contagion to your advantage. The secret to successfully adopting a healthy lifestyle is not willpower, but to be part of a positive social network. Make sure you have social scaffolding and coping mechanisms in place before you attempt a lifestyle change. Associate with friends who want the same lifestyle. Join a club or group activity that is oriented towards the same objective as yours. And avoid unnecessary events where you know the social pressure will detract from your objective.

It is really important to be part of, and contribute to, the right tribe. Finding the right tribe will mean you will not only be able to achieve more, but you will also benefit from increased health and longevity.

CHAPTER TWELVE: SUCCESSFUL AGEING

This chapter is relevant to everyone, not just those of advancing years. Unfortunately the inescapable fact is none of us are getting out of here alive. Whichever way you look at it, we get old and then we die. We have no control over the passing of time, but thankfully we do have a large degree of influence over how successfully we age. Gerontology research suggests that we have between 75 and 80 percent control over how well we age, the remainder being down to our genetics. Successful ageing is about maximising lifespan whilst maintaining vitality for as long as possible, a concept known as healthspan.

HEALTHSPAN

It is generally accepted, often expected, that from middle age onwards we become increasingly unfit, unhealthy and unattractive. It is a given that when we are old we can expect to suffer impairment and fragility. At a time when they have no dependents, no mortgage and an abundance of free time, many pensioners live with the irony of having no vitality to take advantage of their enviable position.

However, this Western version of ageing is not the only version. Let us use blood pressure as an example. In the UK and the USA around one in three adults have high blood pressure, a condition known as hypertension. Hypertension is an independent health risk factor. After the age of forty the prevalence of hypertension increases with advancing age, with around sixty percent of adults suffering from the condition once they reach 65 years. Yet if we examine the blood pressure of people living pre-industrial lifestyles, such as the San Bushmen, we see that for the vast majority their blood pressure remains within normal limits throughout their lives. This trend is similar for other markers of health too. Many elderly Western people suffer chronic illnesses that are not products of ageing per se, but are the result of a lifetime of poor health choices. Making good lifestyle choices now, no matter what your age, will pay dividends later on by increasing your healthspan.

YOU ARE TOO OLD NOT TO

Chronological age is often used as a self-diagnostic tool to provide a reason for failure at a particular activity, or it is used as an excuse to not even try it in the first place. 'I'm too old for that,' is the reasoning and it is further reinforced by a partisan society. Poor strength and mobility, weak bones and joints, and an ailing cardiovascular system are simply regarded as part of the normal ageing process.

To provide proof positive, if a sedentary older person attempts a strenuous activity and becomes injured as a result, it serves to reinforce the previous assumptions that older people should not perform such an activity and that they should return to their sedentary ways. However, it need not be so. It is not necessarily the fault of age per se. In this example, the aetiology of the injury had a temporal component, but it may have been distinct from age. By this I mean it is more likely that the length of time spent living an unhealthy life that was the culprit. It just so happened that the individual got older while the effects manifested. In this instance, the injury likely occurred due to insufficient strength and conditioning for the activity, not because of how many birthdays had passed. Remember structure and situation from Chapter Six? It applies to everyone, no matter their age.

Nonetheless in our modern, mostly sedentary population it is well documented that age is an independent risk factor with regard to health. Therefore it is imperative that before making any lifestyle changes - even positive ones - you take heed of the DISCLAIMER at the beginning of this book and you seek advice from your General Practitioner, Physician or medical professional to determine your suitability for a lifestyle change, this is especially so if you have made poor health choices in the past.

A definitive understanding of the process of ageing does not exist. In part, this is due to ageing being a multifactorial concept, and coupled with methodological difficulties it makes performing longitudinal research on humans problematic. As such a lot of studies focus on ageing in non-human animals as they tend to have more compact lifecycles. For obvious reasons, caution should be exercised when transposing the findings from this type of research to humans. Nonetheless, taking these issues into account, a strong theme amongst the research becomes apparent; the fitter the organism is, the longer it tends to live.

Conventional wisdom would have us believe that our fitness attributes decrease considerably with age; strength, aerobic capacity, power and mobility are all on the decline. The only things that typically increase as we get older are body fat and reaction time, both of which are nothing to brag about! But it is a serious issue. Exercise capacity as a whole is a major predictor for the incidence of death; as your exercise capacity reduces so too do your healthspan and your lifespan.

Sure, there is going to be an inevitable reduction in health and fitness over time, and to date no one has managed to cheat death. But the rate of decline need not be anywhere near as steep as we typically observe or expect. There are outliers in our communities we are all familiar with: those pensioners who have a work rate of someone half their age, or those sports stars who are competing at world-class levels at an age that is well beyond the norm. Are they really outliers, or are these merely examples of what is achievable with correct lifestyle choices?

Of the few longitudinal studies investigating the effects of exercise on ageing in humans, most have found that those who begin regular exercise at a young age and continue it throughout their lives do see a decline in fitness after about 50 years of age, but the subsequent year-on-year reduction is barely noticeable. The fitness levels of these older cohorts are often just as good as (if not better than) those of 20 year olds who do not exercise.

Born-again exercisers (those who take up regular exercise later in life) have also been shown to benefit from a reduced rate of decline albeit from a lower starting point than the lifelong exercisers. Interestingly the born-again exercisers often benefit from an initial increase in their health and fitness markers, in effect reversing the so-called ageing process for a period. The sedentary elderly have a lot to gain from engaging in exercise as they have the most to reclaim.

Preventative maintenance

A year old car may still look new, but it is not. The inevitable degradation has already begun. Unseen parts have begun wearing out, gaskets and seals have started perishing and corrosion has begun taking hold. But it still looks new. Then one day a threshold is crossed. A rust bubble appears on the wheel arch, or the brakes feel spongy, or an oil patch is noticeable on the driveway. Yesterday all seemed fine, but today something is wrong. We can extend this analogy to ourselves, maybe in our twenties we look young and healthy and free from disease, and we can bounce back from reckless lifestyle choices seemingly with impunity. But the effects of ageing are accumulating behind the scenes. Then one day something appears wrong. In a similar way that we can reduce the effect of wear and tear on a car by looking after it, so too can we reduce the rate of degradation of our health as we get older.

Muscular strength, aerobic capacity and mobility are health components as well as being fitness ones. If they are neglected and atrophy over time, there will be a concomitant functional decline in health. Being sedentary is therefore an age accelerant; nearly a third of deaths from heart disease, colon cancer and diabetes are attributed to insufficient physical activity. Maintaining these health components is important as we get older. In Chapter Four we noted that exercise, in the form of resistance training, developed all of these health components, so it is therefore an essential tool for ameliorating the ageing process. Furthermore, the ideal weekly physical activity profile (Figure 4, Chapter Four) maintains its relevance as we get older. A lot of the symptoms that we associate with ageing can be lessened and may even be reversed as a result of exercise. If the rate of degradation of our health and fitness attributes are the telltale signs of ageing, then it follows that exercise is currently the closest thing we have to an elixir of youth.

Muscular strength is perhaps one of the main casualties we associate with getting older. It does not seem to matter what culture we come from - be it Western or hunter and gatherer - after the age of forty we tend to lose muscle mass. This age-related muscle loss is known as sarcopenia, and for Western adults it can be as much as eight percent with each passing decade. After the age of 75 the rate of loss increases rapidly. Recently published longitudinal research has found that in a large cohort of over 50s those who had low levels of muscle strength had twice the likelihood of dying within twenty years compared with those who had normal levels of muscle strength. But before you despair, it is important to note that these are observations from our modern, mostly sedentary population; we do not observe the same rate of strength decline in hunters and gatherers or the active.

Yes, sarcopenia is real, but the high rate at which it occurs in Western adults is more likely a result of the increase in sedentary behaviour as they get older. Research on runners in their 70s and 80s have shown they have similar bone and muscle mass to those in their 40s. It is now widely accepted that muscular strength has a protective effect on mortality, thus by engaging in resistance exercise we can reduce the age-related loss in muscle strength and extend our healthspan.

In Figure 4, Chapter Four we noted it is important to perform some short-duration vigorous physical activity each week. Research is showing that brief occasional bursts of vigorous exercise trigger a host of beneficial effects, including hormonal responses and positive gene expression that promote successful ageing. This brief vigorous activity provides a protective and anabolic effect on lean muscle, it increases mitochondria and energy production, it improves blood lipid ratios and insulin sensitivity, and it increases mental awareness.

Typically, after 50 years of age maximal aerobic capacity (a marker of cardiovascular fitness) declines by 1.5 percent per year. Thankfully research is showing that being active has a protective effect on the rate of this decline and can reduce it to a third of that observed in sedentary individuals. It is also worth noting that for lifelong exercisers this decline also begins from a higher starting point. At all ages the aerobic capacity of the active is around 25 percent better than their sedentary counterparts.

TOO MUCH OF A GOOD THING

In the pursuit of comfort we have outsourced a lot of our physical stress to machines and in doing so reduced the stimulus for optimal self-repair. Davis's law is the physiological principle that tissue is modelled according to the demands imposed on it. We know that muscles get bigger from the stress of contracting against a resistance and that bones get denser as a result of repeated load-bearing impact (the leg bones of runners are denser than those of their sedentary counterparts). We also know that sarcopenia and osteoporosis (the loss of bone mass) are associated with ageing. Clearly if we are sedentary and do not apply sufficient stress to our muscles and bones then we are hastening the rate of ageing. This is one of the prices to pay for a comfortable lifestyle. To a large extent hunters and gatherers do not age in the Western sense. They are active, capable humans for their entire lives save a short deterioration period at the end. In contrast, our comfortable ways have meant we age early and are sick for a protracted period.

Fewer calories, more life

Consuming too many calories is not only bad for your waistline, but also your health. In particular eating too much leads to obesity which in turn predicates a plethora of metabolic disorders and reduces life expectancy.

In addition, there is a growing body of evidence showing that calorie restriction extends the lifespan of mammals (typically mice, there is a paucity of research on humans) for reasons independent of obesity. Overeating has been linked to premature ageing, and suggested causes range from interfering with how genes work to disrupting circadian rhythms. Whilst the effects of calorie restriction and better ageing are observable, the exact mechanisms are not yet fully understood. Until there is more evidence for a demonstrable benefit to humans it is probably not advisable to reduce your calorie intake if you are at your ideal weight, however it does strengthen the argument to consume less if you are overweight. Interestingly, it also suggests that the Okinawan centenarians of Japan are perhaps onto something with their practice of hara hachi bu, "eat until you are 80 percent full."

Deal with it

A key determinant of successful ageing is acceptance. Senescence, the process of cellular deterioration with age, is a natural process and despite even the most ardent efforts will still occur no matter what. It is an immutable fact that you are going to age. Gerontology research consistently shows that those who are happy with their ageing age better. Ageing happens to everyone and refusing to accept it is to fight a losing battle that will ironically only serve to expedite the ageing process. Rather than focus on what you are losing, be positive about your future and the benefits that await you.

As we have seen in the previous chapter, our social network influences how we think and behave. If you hang around with people who have the established

Western view of ageing then it is going to affect your own view of ageing and in turn have a negative influence on how you age. If you really want to maximize your healthspan, you must have the outlook of a younger person, and reject the standard attitude of the old. If you associate with those who have a positive view of ageing you will think and behave like them. Keep a lookout for older mentors or role models who buck the trend and do not conform to the accepted model of decrepitude with advancing years. Seek out those with a young spirit, healthy body and passion for life. There are plenty out there. Follow them on social media and be inspired by them.

The older you get the less your chronological age matters, and the more your biological age comes into play. Most people in their early twenties have a similar biological age. Typically, when we are in our thirties the bifurcation between chronological and biological age begins to show, and then can magnify considerably with each passing decade. For people in their seventies, their biological ages can differ tremendously. You cannot do anything about your chronological age, so do not get hung up on the number. You do however have control over your biological age. No matter where your starting point is, aim to be the best you can be at your current age.

In one respect ageing can be viewed as a battle between your body's ability to maintain itself and the environment in which it exists. The rate at which you lose ground in this battle determines the rate at which you age. Estimates vary, but some experts suggest that we can realistically expect to add a decade of quality time to our lives and compress the degenerative phase to a minimum at the end. An extended life is of little use if you are not feeling good and enjoying these extra years. Successful ageing is dependent on the interaction of a multitude of lifestyle choices. Your choices. Making healthy choices now will increase your chances of independence and enjoyment well into old age.

Thank you for purchasing this book and supporting my work. If you enjoyed it, please leave an online review. For more health and fitness information be sure to follow me on Instagram (johnmetcalfecoaching) and subscribe to my YouTube channel (johnmetcalfecoaching). For enquiries about online health and fitness consultation, please email me (johnmetcalfecoaching@gmail.com).

John

ABOUT THE AUTHOR

John Metcalfe is a health and fitness coach, physical educator and award-winning writer. He first began exercising over 35 years ago and it has been his lifelong passion ever since. He has pursued an academic career in the field of sport, exercise and nutrition science for over 25 years. During this time John has distilled his theoretical understanding and his personal experience into a minimalistic and sustainable healthy lifestyle. Reclaim Your Vitality encapsulates how John lives his healthy life.

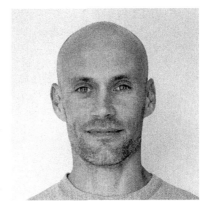

INDEX

INDEX

Printed in Great Britain
by Amazon

83264079R00088